The Healing Power of Light and Color

Colophon

The healing power of light and color
A practical guide to colorpuncture according to Peter Mandel

Originally published as: De verborgen kracht von licht en kleur, Amsterdam, 2013

Author: Praveeta Timmerman, co-writer: Anurago Frese
Translation: Anurago Frese (Fretext)
Published by Esogetics, Bruchsal, Germany

Design cover: Hans-Juergen Mandel, Graphik & Layout

1st edition 2014
2nd edition 2018
3rd edition 2026

The quotes from Peter Mandel are used with permission.

Hildastr. 8 • D-76646 Bruchsal
info-de@esogetics.com • www.esogetics.com
Tel: +49 (0) 7251 80010

DISCLAIMER
In compiling this book the greatest care has been taken to the accuracy of the information contained herein. Some diseases or conditions are not, or less, suitable for self-medication. Always consult your doctor or specialist. The author and publisher of this book are in no way responsible for any injury or consequences arising from the use of this book.

ISBN 978-3-925806-63-6

THE HEALING POWER OF LIGHT AND COLOR

A practical guide to colorpuncture
according to Peter Mandel

Praveeta Timmerman

together with
Anurago Frese

Esogetics GmbH

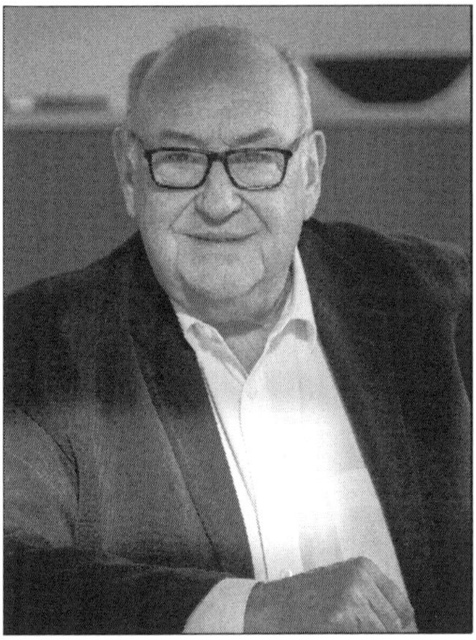

Preface

When I started developing colorpuncture in 1977, I could not imagine that 35 years later this new form of therapy would have spread around the globe. In those days introducing new energetic methods of treatment within the existing medical system was not a matter-of-course. I had to endure much rejection and ridicule in the early days. Paradigm shifts in physics as well as in medical science has changed all of that. Thanks to quantum physics a new medical science has evolved in which new fields were created leading to an increasing understanding of the foundation of all that is alive.

The information of light and colors, combined with a flow of energy, can regulate the vibrating cells that have lost their natural function, because these cells are ultimately formed by light and light frequencies. Without light there is no life and because the frequencies of light – the colors – correspond to the functions of our cells and organs, colorpuncture is not only extremely effective in healing the sick, but also can be a preventive measure for the healthy.

The author of this book, my dear friend Praveeta Timmerman, started her training with me 20 years ago. Nowadays she shares the knowledge she has attained around the world. From a trainee she developed into a teacher. Based on her own personal experience, her clinical observation in her practice over the years, the success of the treatments that she witnessed in the patients entrusted to her care, she now teaches others the basics of colorpuncture. The great merit of Praveeta Timmerman is her capability of integrating the knowledge she has attained, developing it further and passing it on.

This book is the result of her personal experience, her enthusiasm and her commitment over the years. I am very happy that she passes on the method of colorpuncture as a means to increase the well-being of everyone.

Peter Mandel

Introduction

Boudhanath, Nepal, about 35 years ago
While traveling in Asia I spent some time in a Buddhist monastery in Nepal where I participated in a one month meditation course. Early in the morning we took breakfast in silence as usual. The sun rose between the mountain tops. I ate my breakfast slightly absent-minded when suddenly the sun shook me and woke me up. That was how I experienced it. The sun rays touched my heart and seemed to give me a message: 'Be aware – I am also here for you.' I really heard the sun say that and I looked around to see if anyone else had heard, seen or felt it. All the others were sitting there in the same way as before. For me it was a transforming moment. The meditations seemed to have opened something in me, enabling me to be deeply touched. Was it the sun or the light? I didn't pay much attention to it at the time, but many years later, when I had become involved with colorpuncture, this memory suddenly surfaced. I can still feel it in my heart, that the light entered me at that moment and woke me up.

Many years after this journey I felt the need for a new direction in my life. I wanted to help people to relax more, to improve their health and I also wanted to give them a taste of consciousness and meditation. Meanwhile my own spiritual journey had led me to Osho, the Indian mystic who has a well-known meditation center in Pune, India. During one of my visits to the Osho Meditation Resort I heard about a training in colorpuncture that was offered there. I knew immediately that this was what I was looking for and applied. I completed the entire training course.

The founder of colorpuncture is the German naturopath Peter Mandel, who came to Pune himself during my training. I met an inspired man, who taught us how to help people with colored light. His message still resonates in me: 'There is no physical complaint without a psychological or emotional factor.' I had learned this already in the training, but when I heard him say it, it touched me deeply. The most fascinating aspect of his method for me is that the body is used as a vehicle to help clear the mind and increase our level of consciousness. This is also an essential element in the Osho meditations and therapy groups – this obvious connection between emotions and physical tensions.

Over the years I connected with Peter Mandel regularly during the seminars and trainings he gave. I was impressed by his drive to disclose the healing properties of light and color, to reach out to more people in order to help them. The success he has with his treatments never fails to encourage me. His method is simple and can be applied at home. Treatment with light and color doesn't have any negative side effects, it is totally clean and no medication is used. His ability to see connections and links which others don't perceive is also truly impressive, such as the correlation between physical symptoms and psychological causes.

Meanwhile I have practiced colorpuncture in Amsterdam for 20 years and I give courses, workshops and professional trainings. I am still excited and touched when I witness the positive effect the treatments have on my clients and how they gain more insight in their situation.

When a client comes to my practice with a physical or emotional complaint, I first ask him/her to give me an overview of the complaints and sicknesses in his or her life. I then take a kirlian photo of the fingers and toes, which shows me the energetic state of the client at the moment. The client lies down on the table and I start the treatment with light and color. I ask him/her to feel the actual complaint and to observe in which part of the body tension is felt. While I shine the light on certain points I may say: 'Let the light go to that part of the body and watch which image or feeling comes up. How is it connected to your complaint?' Usually there is such a connection. The points I treat with colored light are related to the complaint and the light helps the client to see more clearly what the complaint is connected to. After the treatment I take another kirlian photo as a control picture, which shows me the effect of the treatment. Sometimes I give homework so that the client may continue the treatment at home.

In this book I shall explain how you can help yourself, your family and friends to create a state of balance by using light and color. Most treatments I describe are easy to apply and don't take much time. Much attention is also given to Peter Mandel's views on sickness and health. My own experience of 20 years has convinced me that this work with light and color can instigate profound changes in life. It can literally lighten up your life. Light and color not only have a healing and harmonizing effect on the body, but can also create more space and freedom on the mental plane. I am happy to pass some of my knowledge and experience on to you.

I hope you enjoy reading and using this book.

Many thanks are due to Osho who taught me to find the light inside myself and to Peter Mandel who taught me how to use light and color for healing.

> *'We are born of light, we live in light, we die in light – we are made out of light. This has been one of the greatest insights of the mystics of all the ages... Now science not only says that man is made of light but that everything is made of light, all is made of electrons, electricity. Science has come to this understanding from a very very long route. The objective route is a very long route; the subjective route is very easy, the shortest possible, because you have only to look within.'*
>
> *Osho*

Praveeta Timmerman

Light is color

Why are leaves green, flowers red, yellow or blue and why are clouds white?

In our childhood we all asked our parents these questions, but do we know the answer ourselves?

Colors exist as the result of light. Color is light and light is color. When it is dark, we don't see colors. The physicist Isaac Newton discovered in the 17th century that the white light of the sunrays can be split into different colors by letting the light pass through a prism. In this way the color spectrum also perceived in the rainbow is visible. Each color has a different frequency or wavelength. The light that falls on a surface is partly absorbed and partly reflected. Our eyes register this as color. The refraction of light in a color spectrum can also be observed in an oil slick, a soap bubble or in the feathers of birds such as peacocks or pheasants.

Our eyes can only see a certain part of the light spectrum, the range between 780 (red) and 400 (violet) nanometer. We cannot see ultraviolet, infrared, X-rays and cosmic rays.

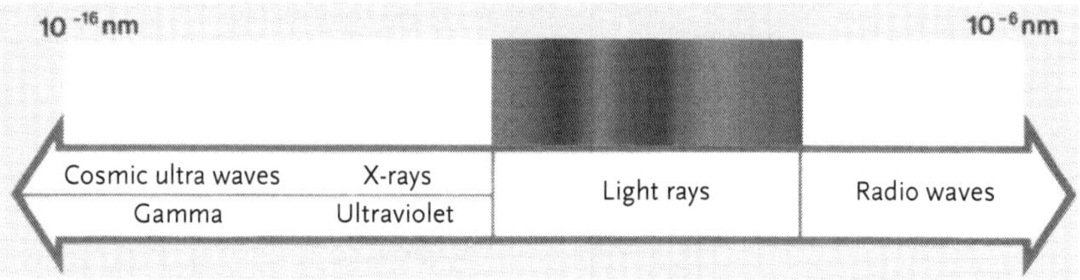

1 *Foundations of light and color*

Light is energy

We live thanks to the sun. Without the light of the sun there would be no life on earth. During the day we are nurtured by the light of the sun and of course by food that grows through sunlight. In the evening, when we have absorbed enough light and have been active, we rest in the dark. That is the balance between yin and yang as described by the Chinese theory of energy. Yin represents the female, receiving principle, rest, relaxation. Yin is also night, the absence of light. Yang is the male principle, action, activity, all that happens in daylight. Yin and yang should be in balance. Every activity should be followed by relaxation. When we sleep, our body regenerates and recovers from the efforts of the day. We could call sleep a 'passive activity'.

We all know very well how deeply light influences our emotional life. On a sunny morning we have no trouble getting up, we are in a good mood and look forward to the day ahead. On a dreary, grey morning we tend to turn over and sleep in. 'Look at the sunny side', we tell someone who is down. Someone who feels depressed craves for more light, wants to come out of the dark tunnel. Seasonal affective disorder (SAD), also called winter depression, can be made 'lighter' by the use of daylight lamps. There are countless examples to show how our inner world of emotions and feelings reacts to light.

Light is the cradle of life. That is also the message many religions give us. The Indian mystic Osho says: "We are born of light, we live in light, we die in light – we are made out of light. This has been one of the greatest insights of the mystics of all the ages."

The Bardo – the Tibetan book of the Dead – as well as modern researchers, e.g. Elisabeth Kübler-Ross, describe the process of dying as a journey towards the light. In mystic traditions human life is often called a journey from darkness to light.

Our cells communicate via light

Dr. Fritz-Albert Popp of the University of Kaiserslautern in Germany discovered in the 1970s that living cells radiate light. He called these light particles biophotons. His research showed that these photons pass on information to other cells by means of light. This light in each cell is extremely weak, but can be measured with special instruments. Popp and his team of researchers conducted tests in which the photon emission of greenhouse tomatoes was compared with that of organically grown tomatoes. The outcome was that organically grown tomatoes emitted twice as many photons! When he compared organic farm eggs with eggs from battery hens, he also found a double emission rate. That makes you think, because that means that organic and naturally grown food could give us extra light and therefore extra energy. If we don't just count calories, vitamins, proteins and minerals in our food intake, but also consider the light and energy stored in our food, we would approach our daily meals in a different way. The processing of fast food and ready-made meals, as well as the storage and additives, also disrupt the coherence of the photons, which results in a lower content of light and life energy in our food.

Popp showed that cells communicate by light. In colorpuncture, developed by the German naturopath Peter Mandel, the emission of light by cells and their communication by means of light is used in two ways, for analysis and to treat diseases. I use the same analytic method in my own practice. A kirlian photo that shows the weak electromagnetic emission of the finger tips and the toes, is made of each client.

The image of the radiation gives me a first impression of the energetic state of health of the client at the moment and allows me to make a first analysis. I then apply colored light on certain points on the skin to improve the energy balance in the body. The name colorpuncture

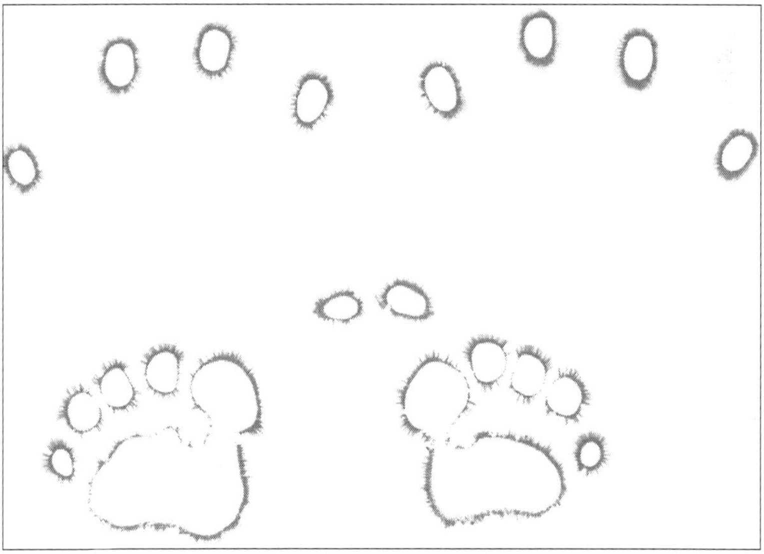

2 *Kirlian photo*

already indicates that light and color are used on acupuncture points, but not exclusively – also on points and zones or lines that were discovered by Peter Mandel over the years. In the past forty years Peter Mandel has developed a wide range of treatments with light and color. In this book I present a selection of treatments that are suitable for self-help at home.

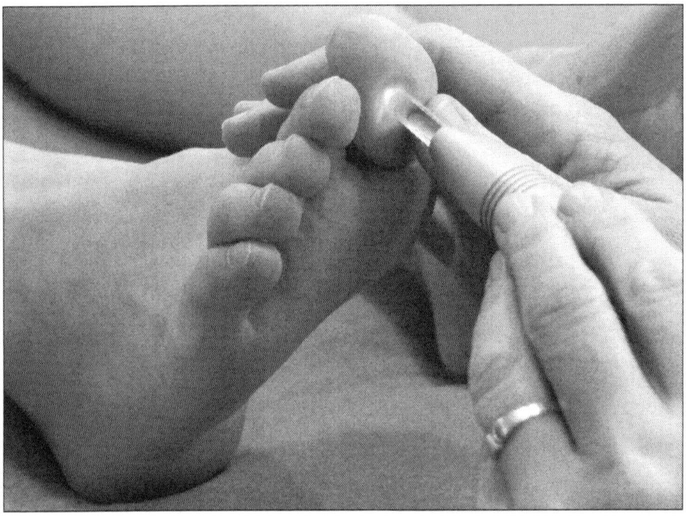

First of all I want to give you some information about colors and their effect.

Colors are carriers of information

The color theory of Goethe is over two centuries old – his book *Farbenlehre* was published in 1810 – but is still regarded as authoritative. He was the first to describe the effects of colors on feelings, their interrelatedness and workings. The primal colors are red, yellow and blue. The other colors are compositions, derived from combinations of the primal colors. Red mixed with yellow gives orange. In this way the complementary colors are formed – they are each other's counterparts: blue has orange as its counterpart, yellow has violet and red has green as its complementary color.

Peter Mandel added turquoise to the three primal and the three complementary colors. Turquoise does not have a complementary

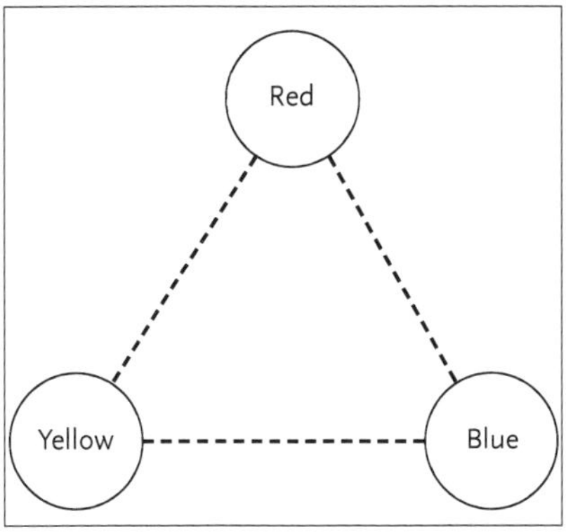

3 *Primary colors*

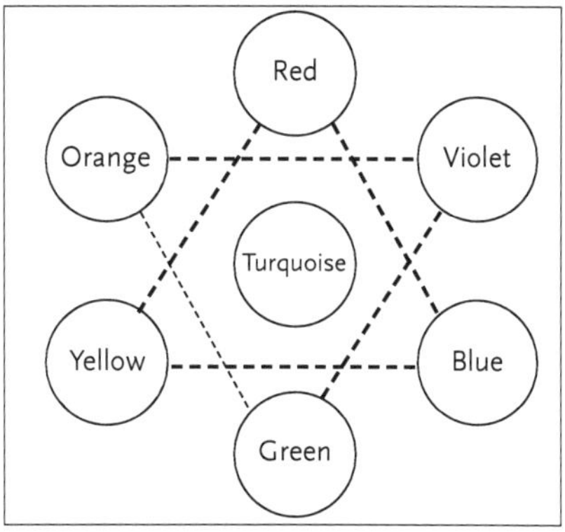

4 *Primary and complementary colors*

color. In his practice this color proved to be the color that influences the subconscious part of the spirit – it is the color of the soul.

The main properties of the seven main colors are described in the chart on the next page.

There are two shades of turquoise – a darker, spectral shade and the lighter 'soul-spirit' shade. The darker shade belongs to the seven chakra or rainbow colors and is often used in colorpuncture.

Colorpuncture therapists also use other colors in their practice that are not explained in this book. These are the so-called soul-spirit colors: light turquoise, light green, crimson and pink. There are also three grey colors, ultraviolet (370 nm) and infrared (950 nm). Ultraviolet and the grey colors are used for disorders with an emotional background. Infrared is used mainly to alleviate pain. In the colorpuncture therapist training the meaning and usage of all these colors are taught.

How can light and color work as healing agents?

Peter Mandel answers this question as follows: "If our organism emits light, then it is obvious for me that it also can absorb light – at the same points. It was an intuition, at first. But in the meantime I have been proven right by a Chinese physicist who showed that the energy

Color chart

COLOR	Effect	Use	Organs	Qualities
RED	Warm color with the strongest power of penetration, stimulates the blood circulation	Weak blood circulation, chronic cough, asthma, anemia, eczema	Heart, lungs, kidneys, bladder, muscles	Love, anger, joy. The choleric temperament
BLUE	Cool color, helps to relax	Alleviation of pain, sleep disorders, impotence, menopause, headache, hemorrhoids, infections, fever, restlessness	Pituitary, endocrine system, muscle cramps, tendons, tissue	Rest, peace, gentleness. The melancholic temperament
YELLOW	Effects the nervous system, digestion, makes chronic processes acute	Digestive problems, lymphatic complaints, weak nervous system	Liver, stomach, spleen, large intestine	Intelligence, understanding, cheerfulness. The sanguine temperament
GREEN	Neutralizing, relaxes organs, detoxifying	Arthritis, tumors, ulcers, cysts, eye diseases, diabetes	Lungs, kidneys, bladder	Satisfaction, relaxation, harmony. The phlegmatic temperament
ORANGE	Gives energy, joy, strength	Depression, anxiety, arteriosclerosis, anorexia, anemia	Heart, small intestine	Joy, happiness, cheerfulness
VIOLET	Stimulates consciousness and intuition, regulates feelings	Lymphatic complaints	Spleen, large intestine, stomach	Meditation, intuition, spirituality
TURQUOISE	Represents the outside of the soul, as it presents itself to the outside world	Emotions that express itself as bodily complaints, psychosomatic diseases	No specific organs	Liberation, wholeness

meridians are in fact light transmitters. In a way the skin is a 'seeing organ'. After all, we virtually live on light, and our body is continuously busy decoding and translating all sorts of exact messages in order to function. We can break down these messages to individual colors. In other words, you shine a particular color onto a point related to a particular organ or brain function. The skin point is linked through meridians – not necessarily the acupuncture meridians – with the target zone inside the body, and the message is transmitted. Color is life energy carrying information. The information heals, and the energy carries the healing information through the cells. This way you can actually reach to the very root of a problem in the brain."

It was well-known in ancient times that light and color have a healing influence. Some temples in ancient Egypt contained rooms where the sick were treated with colored light. In Greece Herodotus developed heliotherapy, a method of treating patients with sunlight. Early in the 20th century scientists discovered that bone-deforming rickets in children was caused by a deficit of vitamin D and that sunlight helped to cure it. That is quite understandable, because we now know that sunlight on the skin helps the body to produce this vitamin. Denmark's Niels Finsen won the 1903 Nobel Prize for his discovery that sunlight could heal skin tuberculosis.

In the 20th century naturopaths often used color and light for healing, but the discovery of antibiotics changed the course of regular medicine. Nowadays it becomes more and more clear that antibiotics and operations, however useful and essential they may be, don't always offer a solution for the diseases of today. Holistic healing methods once again attract attention. Holistic natural healing puts the human being in its totality in the spotlight. It regards man as a unity of body, spirit and soul. Colorpuncture, as developed by Peter Mandel over the past forty years, combines ancient and new insights of both Eastern and Western healing methods into a new form of light therapy.

Give your health a boost with light and color

In daily life you can easily nourish yourself more with light and color. Many people in our society spend most of their time during the day indoors and don't absorb enough sunlight. Our yang energy doesn't get charged enough and we are not as active and vital as we could be. We stay up late, watch TV or spend time on our computer, the lights are on and we absorb too much artificial light, disturbing our yin energy. And if the bedroom is not dark enough, it's no wonder we suffer from insomnia or other sleeping disorders, because our rhythm of light and darkness has been disturbed. Soon this creates a vicious circle – lack of sleep causes us to feel tired during the day, we don't feel fit, body and mind are out of sync, which makes us lie awake at night. It is very important that we all absorb more daylight in order to strengthen our yang energy. We can also do ourselves a favor by sleeping in a dark bedroom – let the nights be really dark – and by spending less time in the evening in front of our TV-set or computer screen. Here are some practical tips that you'll find easy to incorporate in your life:

- Ensure you have a good day/night rhythm. Don't spend too much time watching TV or working on the computer in the evenings.
- Be outdoors for at least half an hour or better one hour daily. Walk or cycle in nature.
- Eat plenty of fresh fruits and vegetables, preferably organic, and make your meals colorful with orange pumpkin, green broccoli, white cauliflower, violet eggplant, red capsicum and tomatoes, orange carrots, red beetroot, blue berries.
- Wear bright, cheerful colors, avoid black or grey in your clothing.
- If you need to spend much time indoors during the day, you can install full spectrum lights in your house or work environment. They provide you with a better light quality.
- If you spend much time on the computer, consider wearing protective computer glasses. They filter out the high quantity of blue light that the screen emits.
- Orange glasses help you if you have a tendency to be depressed or sad. The orange color gives you a big dose of zest for life. You can find information on color glasses in the last section of this book.

And how about the colors of flowers and plants?

The colors of the flowers developed during evolution through an interaction between the plant and its environment. Plants could propagate with the help of insects who were attracted by colors and smells and were in return rewarded with honey. The insect carries the pollen and spreads it when visiting other flowers. This pollination by insects is highly effective and has a wider range than pollination by wind alone.

Why are leaves green and why do flowers have beautiful colors? Light contains all the colors of the rainbow. The green parts of the plants have a light absorbing pigment named chlorophyll, that absorbs red and blue light. These parts only reflect green light and that's why we see them as green. If we look at the leaf of a plant through a microscope, we see small green granules in the leaf cells, called chloroplasts. This is where the chlorophyll molecules are located. Chlorophyll is a catalyst. It uses the solar energy to bring about a chemical reaction that helps the plant to get its energy. This chlorophyll conversion provides to a large extent the energy that is available for us on this planet.

Instead of chlorophyll other pigments are made in the flowers of plants, that give them their striking colors. Depending on the species, the plant carries red, yellow or orange pigments in its genes. These pigments cause the flowers to have different colors. Pigments are small granules which are responsible for the reflection of light rays. Red pigments reflect the red light spectrum. Our human eyes see different colors than insect eyes. Bees can see ultraviolet light (beyond blue and violet), that we are not able to see.

Ancient traditional Chinese medicine, that is over 5000 years old, already discovered the effect of colorful flowers on people. Flowers have been used for thousands of years to evoke certain feelings. According to Chinese medicine, the secret lies in the color of the flower. When we perceive a color it in fact means light waves of a certain frequency touch the eye and the retina. The optical nerve in the retina leads the impulses to our brain, which then causes a chain reaction in our body. Neurotransmitters are released that stimulate the production of soothing hormones like melatonin, stimulating hormones such as adrenalin and pleasure inducing hormones such as serotonin.

2

Sickness and health according to Peter Mandel

In this chapter we investigate the way of thinking that is the foundation of therapeutic treatment with light and color. In order to do so we need to leave mainstream allopathic medicine aside for the moment. It often regards people as machines that have a structural defect and need repair. This doesn't mean Peter Mandel rejects regular medical science as such. He says: 'Colorpuncture is not an exclusive healing system. Of course we need allopathy. I cooperate with all the allopathic doctors in my area. It is a matter of mutual support. They help where I can't help and vice versa. Please get that straight: I am not against allopathy – I am against the way it is being used. On the whole, it is being used unconsciously, routinely, even murderously at times, callously, without a deeper commitment to the patient or to the full implications of a given disease. No, where surgery is needed, surgery is needed. The same goes for antibiotics. But these things are not always needed where they are applied.'

Peter Mandel's approach is holistic and closely related to naturopathy. Man is seen as part of nature, as part of the universe. Body, spirit and soul are one. This view corresponds with the ancient Chinese traditional medicine, that regards meridians and acupuncture points as a energetic grid that is found throughout the body. Communication via meridians and points takes place mainly through light (photons), as I mentioned in chapter 1. Impulses of light and color applied to the skin can actually trigger and improve the communication between the living cells.

A new approach to healing

Mandel calls his system 'esogetics' or 'esogetic healing'. The name esogetics is a compound of the words esoteric and energetic. In coining this new term Mandel indicates that this new way of healing incorporates ancient wisdom and the understanding of cosmic laws with bio-energetics and modern biophysics.

The esoteric aspect is the path of inquiring into who we are, an understanding that comes from the soul. This knowing is not logical and can only be found through an inner experience, a seeing that comes from meditation. This path of self-knowledge is open to all, but many people are not ready to take it, because it cannot be understood through the mind or by rational thinking. It requires a giving up of set patterns of behavior and thought. Central to the esogetic model is the statement of the ancient Egyptian mystic Hermes Trismegistos 'as above, so below' – macrocosm reflects microcosm, inside equals outside, the same universal laws govern everywhere. All knowledge is already present in its potential, nothing is really new. An obvious illustration of 'as above, so below' is our solar system, which is replicated in the structure of the atom. Within the atom the electrons orbit around the central nucleus, just as planets revolve around the sun. All discoveries and inventions in science are truly dis-coveries, which are found – a veil, a layer is taken away and reveals something 'new' which was in fact already there.

The energetic aspect is just as important, for we don't exist as pure matter. Without energy, vitality and a flow of information there would be only dead matter and life would not be possible. Modern science too is accepting the fact that energy forms the base of matter. Max Planck already describes matter as a form of energy.

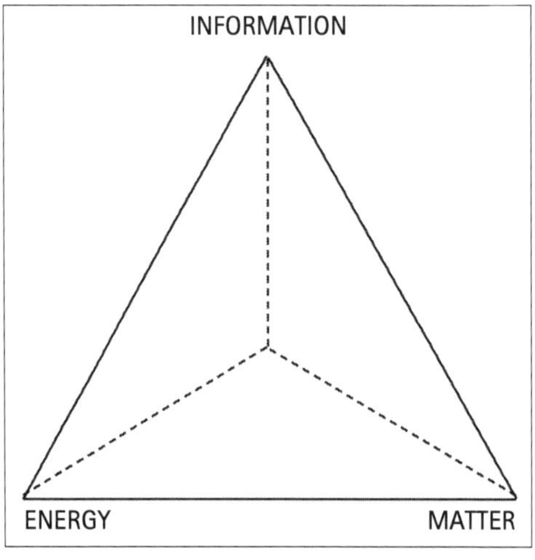

5 *Matter – Energy – Information*

The cells in our body are carriers of information. They execute a inherent program. This information is unique for each one of us. A seed of an oak can never grow into a beech. Each cell in our body is pre-programmed with a matrix and every human being feels from birth a deep desire to follow his own, unique path in life. We all have bones, muscles, nerves, organs, veins, but still each of the billions of humans that inhabit this earth is completely unique and unlike any other human being. Compare just for a moment a human being with a computer. The hardware (matter) is similar in all of us, the computer takes its energy from the power network, but our software (information) is quite individual and specific for each one of us. Energetics deals with this trinity of matter, energy and information.

Why do we get sick?

According to Peter Mandel sickness represents the opposite of health – health being a state of aliveness, activity, joy and creativity. Sickness means frustration and pain, our life force is paralyzed and life energy is not flowing at its optimum. In his practice Peter Mandel encourages his patients to investigate and introspect in order to discover what has caused their sickness. Treatments with light and color help to awaken this insight. The light penetrates to deeper layers of consciousness and brings up pictures or visions that can indicate the cause of the complaint. This requires a shift in the mind-set of the patient as well as the therapist. The local pain or the complaints are no longer the main issue and the focus is no longer on how to solve the symptom. We need to go all the way back in order to find the cause.

The cause is often not directly related to the syndrome of the patient. Quite often conflicts in childhood – which according to Peter Mandel are mostly found around the age of 3, 6, 9 and 12 – are the cause of sickness at a later date, even if we are not conscious of such a conflict, which may lie hidden in the past. Such psychological or physical burdens can haunt people during their whole life and manifest in many varying complaints. Most physical complaints are caused by earlier psychologically testing situations or by acute or chronic conflicts. The complaints can only disappear or diminish if the cause of the sickness is recognized. It is certain that each pain, each sickness has a cause, because everything in life is subject to a process of development and an illness doesn't just fall from the sky.

Every human being needs to follow his individual path in life and has the opportunity to learn from the situations he meets. If he learns and stays on his path in spite of all setbacks, he can be healthy. If he doesn't learn, a sickness will occur. Peter Mandel often gives the example of someone who goes through life with open eyes, but closes them for a moment and immediately lands in a swamp. Of course he jumps out quickly and makes sure he is more aware next time. Someone else may not be so alert and stays in the mud, complains about cold and wet feet, becomes the victim of the situation and starts to blame others for his fate. Soon he will be sick, get a cold, a fever or a pneumonia. He forgets the light, the beauty and purity he had at birth. He only feels the cold in his limbs and gets accustomed to his misery. Well, that's how it is, this is my fate, he thinks. If he is lucky, a friendly neighbor passes by who encourages him to come out of the swamp. If he does so, he can warm his feet and acknowledge that life is beautiful. Maybe he has learned a lesson and will avoid the swamp next time.

Each time we go astray from our path in life, we encounter the consequences as a lesson. Sickness and physical complaints are the first signals. The doctor or therapist should then offer the kind of help that motivates the patient to analyze himself and his surroundings, to discover and remove the cause of his sickness. That requires quite a bit of courage. It is not easy to step out of engrained habits.

We have to be willing to see that all joy and suffering, fear and pain, happiness and frustration don't come from the outside – we create those feelings ourselves. As soon as this is understood there is an opening to reach a true insight and then the process of healing can start. If everyone would understand that we, as individuals, are but a cell in the organism of the earth, we would stop fighting other cells (other people). What happens outside of us, like war and fights, also happens inside of us (cells fighting each other).

Colorpuncture developed by Peter Mandel as a treatment with light and color is not a symptomatic therapy. It doesn't just cure the headache or the skin disease. Its main purpose is to dissolve the blocks in the flow of information inside the body and by doing so remove the cause of pain or dis-ease.

Prevention is better than cure

Of course it is preferable to prevent a latent disease, rather than cure it. We can do that by strengthening our immune system with light and color treatments and by restoring the inner harmony before any symptoms of disease occur. In this book I give you several examples of such preventive treatments, that can easily be done at home with a light set, herbal oil or sound therapy. By giving yourself a simple 10 minute coordination treatment daily in the morning you can start your day in inner harmony and balance. Before going to sleep you can rub esogetic herbal oil on certain points or zones of the body to help you relax and connect with your inner world through dreams. These treatments with light and color are an aid to connect consciously with the innate wisdom of your body. You will pick up warning signals that something is amiss early and you can respond adequately by adjusting your life pattern. There are also treatments for children who are fearful or have trouble learning.

Discovering causal connections

While giving courses and trainings, I often hear participating therapists comment on the fascinating new causal connections Peter Mandel points out, how they offer new insights in the background of the symptoms. A good example is the principle of the 'inverted man' that is often used in Peter Mandels treatments.

We return to the statement of Trismegistos 'as above, so below' that we discussed earlier in this chapter. Peter Mandel took this statement literally and arrived at amazing insights that he tested in his practice during many years before publishing them.

If you fold the image of the human body as if it were a puppet, the head lies in the pelvis. Peter Mandel discovered that he could treat complaints in the pelvis by shining colored light on certain points on the head and that eye complaints could be treated successfully by

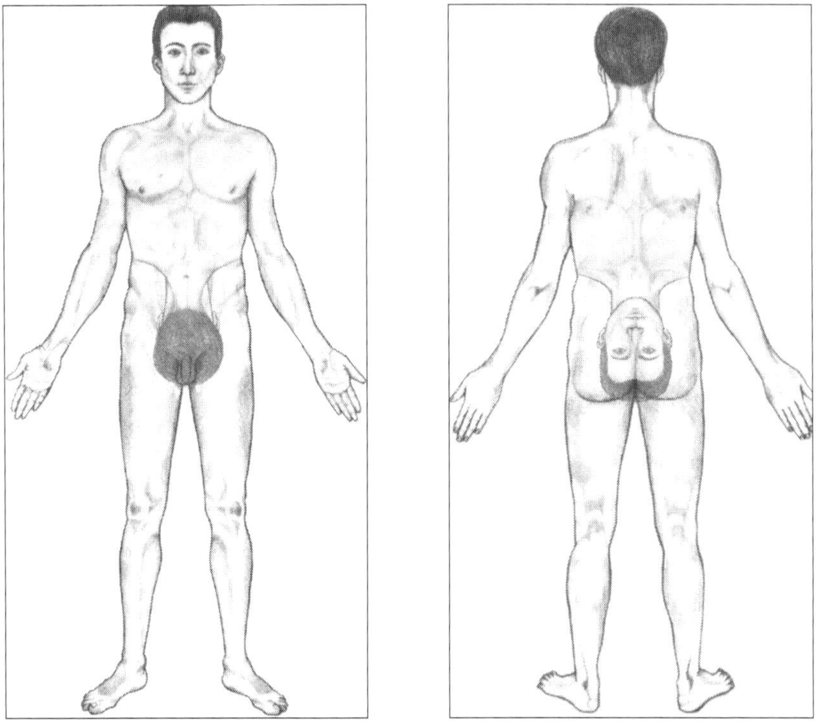

6 *Principle of the inverted man*

radiating points on the lower back. At first this seems strange and unbelievable, but his method proved very successful in his clinic.

According to this principle 'as above, so below' the fingers and toes are also complimentary to each other, connected by invisible energetic lines. These connections are based on the well-known meridians in traditional Chinese medicine and on modern meridians, that were discovered by Dr. Reinhold Voll. The reflex zones on the feet have similar connections.

- Thumbs and big toes both represent the head and also liver, spleen and pancreas.
- Index fingers and second toes are connected to the nervous system, large intestine, joints and stomach.
- Middle fingers and toes relate to the blood circulation, skin and connective tissue.

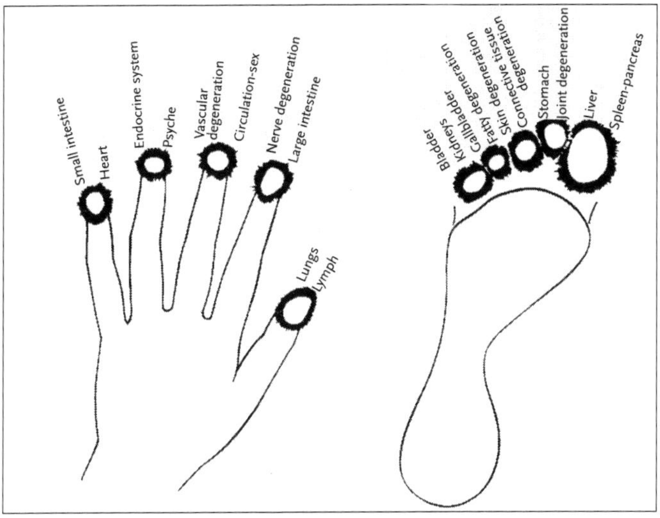

7 *The meridians of the fingers and toes*

- Ring fingers and toes are connected to the hormonal system and digestion of fat (gall bladder)
- Little fingers and toes represent the heart, small intestine, bladder and kidneys.

In chapter 5 you find a harmonizing treatment using colored light on fingertips and toes.

Based on the principle of the inverted man the back of the head, neck and shoulders are connected with the lower belly. Once you see these connections you may notice that many people who have belly problems, also complain about pain in neck and shoulders. I notice in my practice that chronic infections of the facial cavities often coincide with lower back complaints.

Finally I would like to mention the connection between the joints:
- the wrists are connected with the ankles
- the elbows with the knees
- the shoulders with the hips

Clients are often amazed that we treat the elbow to relieve pain in the knee!

An example from my daily practice illustrates this.

> *Anna phoned me to make an appointment because she suddenly had severe lower back pain. When she arrived she could hardly walk, sit or lay down because of the pain. It had started 'out of the blue' yesterday morning. For me 'out of the blue' is always a reason to ask some more questions. I asked her what had happened in her life recently. She told me she had started a new job two months ago and that she found it quite challenging. In the beginning she felt a bit insecure, but it seemed to go quite well, until she got a cold three weeks ago that developed into a sinusitis. She didn't want to report ill at the start of her new career, took some painkillers and continued work, while letting her illness run itself out during the weekends. The sinusitis was not over yet and had bothered her for quite some time now. She didn't want to take more painkillers for her back problem. When I showed her the picture of the inverted man, she suddenly saw the connection. She realized that the pressure at work had caused her cold and that repressing her cold – a toxic reaction of the body that she had failed to take as a signal – now resulted in lower back pain. I treated her cold with colorpuncture and gave her some pain relieving treatment for her lower back. After a few days she felt much better.*

The valuable aspect of colorpuncture according to me is the fact that light and color give an energetic, healing impulse that provides the clients with an insight which helps them to solve their problems by themselves.

When I give a light and color treatment I always ask the clients to look inside and feel what is happening in their bodies and in their lives. Because the light literally 'enters', they can see the dark corners of their inner world – often for the first time. They start to understand why their bodies have gone off course. This 'seeing' is the first step towards healing and change. The pain or the complaint that brings the client to me are signals and as soon as the signal is understood, the pain can leave.

3

Getting off to a good start with colorpuncture

Before you start with colorpuncture and the other suggestions that I give you in the following chapters, I recommend you read this chapter first.

Giving treatments using the light set

In the annex of this book you find a description of two light sets that can be used for giving treatments: the flat focus light set and the light set for point treatment. They can be ordered at www.kleurenpunctuur.nl or www.esogetics.com. If you are a therapist or acupuncturist, I would advise you to use the light set for point treatment. Anyone else is better off using the flat focus set.

The following points are important to observe when giving treatments:

- The flat focus set can be switched on by turning the top of the torch until the light comes on. Put the colored cap on and place the torch in a 90 degree angle on the point that you want to treat.

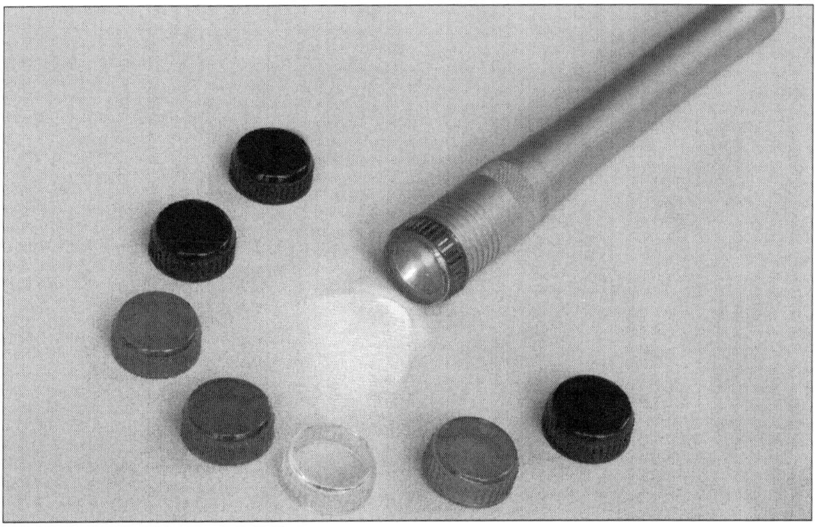

- The light set for point treatment has glass rods. Turn the top of the torch until the light comes on. Stick the glass rod with the colored part into the torch and place the pyramid-shaped end on the point that you want to treat.

- The pyramid-shaped top of the glass rod or the cap of the flat focus light set should touch the skin during the treatment.

- Ask your partner or a friend to help you treat any points or lines on the back of the body that are difficult to reach.

- The sequence of points, zones or lines to be treated are clearly described with each treatment, as well as the duration of the application of the light. It is important to observe these instructions exactly.

- The light is usually applied for 30 seconds on each point, unless otherwise indicated. For children the light is applied for a shorter time – the younger the child, the shorter the treatment per point will be. For small babies this could be only 5 seconds per point.

- Whenever a negative reaction occurs, the treatment of that point stops and you continue to treat the next point. Even babies indicate clearly when they have had enough – they turn away, withdraw their leg or arm. Sometimes you can see them relax, they stop crying or fall into a deep sleep. When that happens the treatment can be stopped, because relaxation has been achieved.

- When two points or zones – left side and right side – need to be treated, you proceed as follows:
  - o If the treatment should be done in the same color, you apply the light first on the point or zone on the left side of the body and then on the right side. By left or right side is meant the left or right side of the client's body.
  - o If you need to use complementary colors, you first test the two points or zones to find which one is more sensitive. Place your thumbs left and right on the points or zones and press lightly. You, or the client, will feel which side is more sensitive or gives more resistance. You can also use the testing rod that is part of the light

set for point treatment. The more sensitive point or zone is treated first with the cool color (blue, violet or green) and then the less sensitive side is given the warm color (orange, yellow or red).

- In the description of the treatments you will find FW = finger width as an indication of distance. A finger width is always the width of the finger of the client. If you treat yourself, you use the width of your own finger. The exact measurement is the width of the middle phalanx of the index finger.

- Often you will find abbreviations of acupuncture points in the descriptions. The location of the point is always clearly given and easy to find, even if you are not familiar with acupuncture points. The abbreviations used are listed in the annex.

- Contraindication: if you suffer from epilepsy or asthma, it is better not to treat yourself, but to contact a colorpuncture therapist in the neighborhood who can give you advice. Most treatments can be applied during pregnancy, but there are point treatments that should be avoided. These are indicated in the treatment description.

- Cleaning: the glass rods and caps can be cleaned with 70% alcohol after use. The glass rods may also be sterilized.

Treatments without a light set

If you don't have a light set at your disposal, you can also treat some of the points by massaging them or rubbing some esogetic herbal oil on them.

Another way to restore the inner balance is by listening to the color-sound therapy CDs. In the next chapters I have indicated which CDs are suitable to support the treatments. The best time to listen to the CDs is late in the afternoon or in the evening before going to sleep.

Color glasses can also give your health and well-being a boost. You will find a reference to color glasses in the description of some treatments.

In the annex you find practical information about esogetic herbal oil, color sound CDs and color glasses.

Getting started

The best way to make use of this book is by hands-on experience. Just start applying the treatments on yourself, your children, friends or family members. Choose the treatment you would like to give and apply it several times in the course of a week – once a day is the maximum. You will personally experience the remarkable effect of light and color. It often needs only one or two treatments to notice a change.

Dr. Pagnamenta, a pediatrician in Switzerland who uses colorpuncture in his clinic, tells the story of the 3-year old Elisa in his book Children in the Light. She had always been terrified of playing on the swing. After one treatment the mother called him to say that Elisa had been on the swing the whole day, with eyes closed and singing happily!

This is, of course, an amazing result, but it is also possible that it takes more time before you or the person you treat feels the effect of light and color. If you notice that the treatment doesn't bring any result after repeating it three to four times, it would be better to make an appointment with a colorpuncture therapist who can advise you about a treatment plan that you can follow at home.

Important disclaimer: Colorpuncture is never an alternative for a thorough medical diagnosis or treatment. Always consult your medical practitioner if you have serious complaints. The treatments in this book are meant for minor complaints, not as home medication for serious illnesses.

This does not mean that colorpuncture, practiced by a certified therapist, could not be of great help for degenerative, serious diseases. Peter Mandel treats countless people daily with light and color in his clinic in Bruchsal, Germany, many of whom were given up by regular medical doctors or hospitals. His success is based on the holistic approach of esogetic medicine. It does not regard a person as purely a compound of biological and physical functions that may be disturbed, but as one entity of body, spirit and soul. Everything we have ever experienced in our life – even before birth – has had an influence on our life up till this very moment. Light and color penetrate to the deepest core of our being, where the cause of the disease is hidden. This cause may be an unresolved childhood trauma, a wrong self-image that you have developed over time or a stack of emotions that have not been dealt with.

When treating yourself pay some attention to which thoughts come up during a treatment or which dreams you have the following night. Some old memories may be stirred up. The same is the case if you treat someone else. Ask the one you treat what thoughts come up and feel at the same time what is happening inside you as you give the treatment. Often the one giving the treatment functions as a mirror for the experiences of the client. I notice again and again that from deep layers of consciousness the answers pop up that are needed to help you on your path in life. It can also be a good idea to keep a diary and note down which treatments you did and what you experienced. Note down your dreams as well, they can give you clear hints which themes are important for you at the moment.

Development of sickness in three stages

4

In this chapter I would like to explain the development of sickness in three stages, as distinguished by Peter Mandel in his system of esogetic holistic medicine. They are the endocrine, the toxic and the degenerative stage. These stages give us an insight in the origin and development of disease. The standard treatments for these three stages support the immune system of the body and are described in this chapter.

The description of each stage shows which one corresponds with your own state of health. You can give yourself or someone else an endocrine or toxic treatment even if you don't feel sick, because they effectively bring your body in balance. The degenerative treatment is more suited for people who suffer from serious, chronic ailments.

In the final chapter of this book I tell more about the degenerative phase and how colorpuncture can help people who have a chronic disease.

The endocrine stage

Stress and tensions cause a slight hormonal imbalance in the body. People's reactions to stress are quite individual. Some get a headache, others a stomach pain or a sleepless night. Medical tests are usually not conclusive, no disease shows up in the tests. The physician probably assumes the cause is psychosomatic. Complaints range from fear, restlessness, headaches, insomnia, stomach or intestinal disorders to hypertension. On the mental plane we notice that people in this stage have doubts whether they have made the right choices in their lives. The endocrine treatment aims at releasing the emotional tension or the stress, restoring the hormonal balance and activating the capacity to relax.

Peter Mandel lists the following complaints as typical for the endocrine stage.

- At the physical level

Hormonal symptoms, causing disturbances in the functioning of organs and physical systems. Usually the symptoms cannot be clinically demonstrated. The often wide range of symptoms include cardiovascular imbalances such as irregular blood pressure, also headaches, restlessness and anxiety, disturbed sleeping patterns or insomnia, dizzy spells, digestive problems, cramps in the stomach area. These people often complain about cold and sweaty limbs, especially about clammy or wet hands. We often see swollen thyroid glands, women with menstrual disorders, and complaints of the stomach and intestinal tract.

- At the level of the soul and the emotions

Here we notice fear, anxiety, mood changes and even depression, which lead to stress and cause a vicious circle. Sometimes there are indications that the stress is related to events in the past, such as a lack of love or intimacy in childhood, unreasonable or physical punishment, separation anxiety. The symptoms can also be related to prenatal stress or birth trauma.

- At the spiritual level

At the spiritual level these people have not been able to fulfill their 'individual program'. They have not yet discovered their own path in life or have lost their way.

THE BASIC ENDOCRINE TREATMENT

The basic endocrine treatment is used to regulate the complaints listed above. This treatment is very effective if you suffer from stress and also helps to dissolve old, emotional tensions from the past. The healing impulses of light and color usually quickly calm down the symptoms and restore the balance.

It is important to observe the sequence of the points. Treat each point for 30 seconds. If unpleasant or negative reactions occur, stop treating that point and continue with the next one.

The abbreviations for the acupuncture points are found in the annex.

Location of the points and sequence:

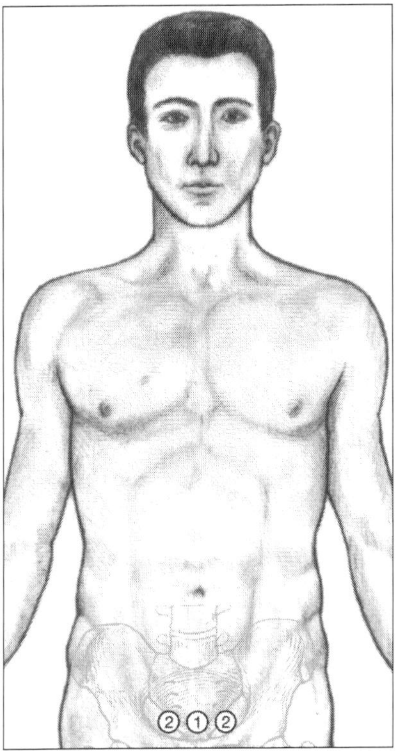

8 *The basic endocrine treatment – 1st step*

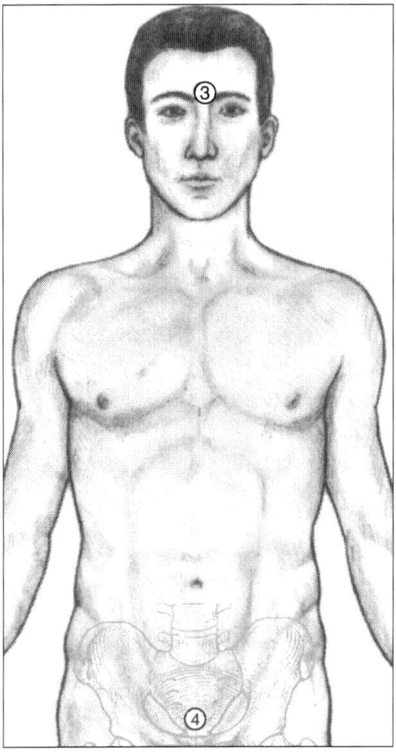

9 *The basic endocrine treatment – 2nd step*

1ST STEP

1 = 1 FW above the edge of the pubic bone, on the middle line .... orange

2 = 2 FW to the left and right of point 1 .... orange

2ND STEP

3 = Yin trang, exactly between the eye brows .... blue

4 = Point 1 .... orange

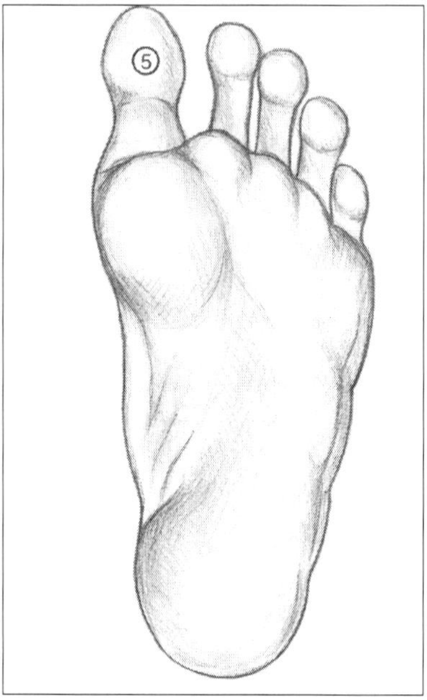

10 The basic endocrine treatment – 3rd step

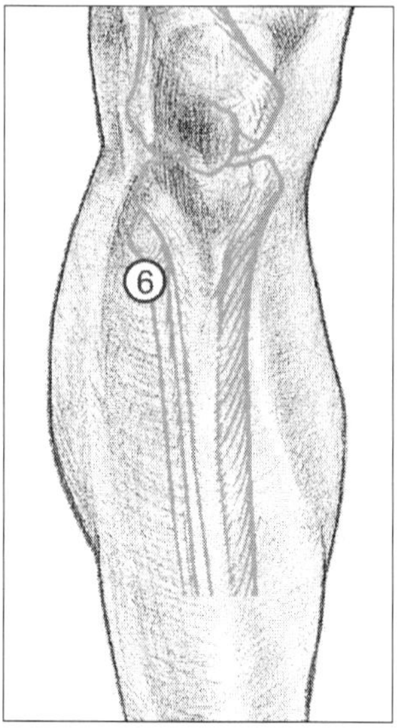

11 The basic endocrine treatment – 4th step

3RD STEP

5 = Pituitary point: in the middle of the big toe, left and right.
Treat with complementary colors .... blue/orange
Test the points for sensitivity. The more sensitive point is treated with blue, the less sensitive point with orange.

4TH STEP

6 = ST 36. Treat complementary .... blue/orange
The more sensitive point with blue, the less sensitive point with orange.

Location of ST 36: this point is found below and to the side of the knee on the outside of the leg. If you put the palm of your hand on your knee (left hand on left knee) and spread your fingers the ring finger lies on this point – it is sensitive to pressure.

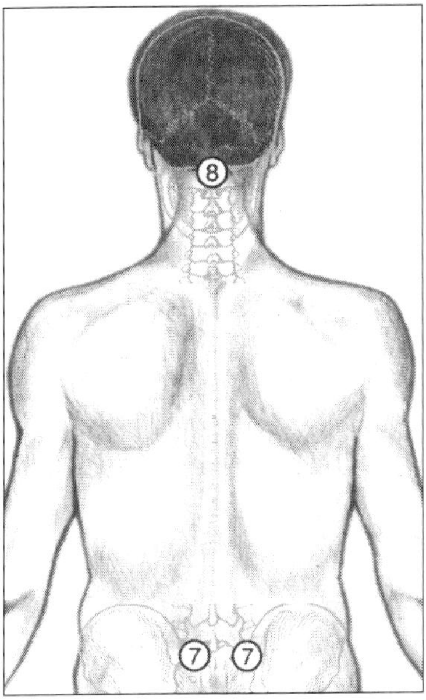

12 *The basic endocrine treatment – 5th and 6th step*

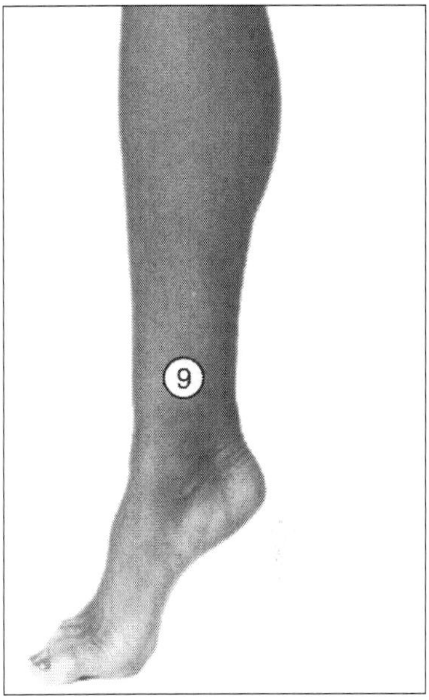

13 *The basic endocrine treatment – 7th step*

5TH STEP

7 = UB 31, first left, then right..red
Location of UB 31: left and right, in the upper hole of the sacrum, 2 FW next to the middle line.

6TH STEP

8 = GV 16. Treat with ....blue
Location of GV 16: under the edge of the skull at the back of the neck, in the middle.

7TH STEP

9 = SP 6, complementary..blue/orange
Location of SP 6: at the outer edge of the tibia, 4 FW above the inside of the ankle bone. Do not treat this point if pregnant!

All points are treated 30 seconds.

The CD Psychosomatic Balance is a good support for this treatment.

The toxic stage

The second stage of development in sickness is the toxic stage. The expression 'toxic' indicates that the body now needs to defend itself against both internal and external toxins or poisons by going into a reaction. At this stage the immune system is already weakened by prolonged stress and hormonal disorder. Infections, allergies, skin rashes, severe fatigue may occur, also sudden pains in the spine and the joints ('I strained my back') belong to this stage.

The treatment of the toxic stage is aimed at stimulating the lymph flow in order to help the body to eliminate waste products. The lymphatic system is responsible for all primary reactions. Mandel regards the lymph as the 'psychological buffer' and calls infections or swellings 'a reaction of the psychological lymphatic buffer'. In the chapter on strengthening the immune system you will find more information about the importance of the lymph and some more treatments for the lymphatic system. The following example shows how an emotionally charged situation can lead to a toxic reaction.

> *A six-year old boy is having lunch with his parents. The parents tell him that they want to go to the theater that evening, but have been unable to find a baby-sitter. That would mean their small son would need to stay at home alone. The father says: 'At your age I also stayed at home alone when my parents went out.' The child is now confronted with the fact that he may have to spend the evening all by himself in this big house. During the afternoon he develops a fever, the lymph nodes in his throat swell up and by the evening he has a severe cold. Of course the parents cancel their visit to the theater. Later that night the boy miraculously recovers and by the morning he is as fit as a fiddle.*

Many parents will recognize this example. It shows that feelings such as fear can create toxic processes. It is quite plausible that this is also the case with other emotional inner conflicts. This example shows us the transition between the endocrine and the toxic stage. The emotional unease seems to grow to such an extent that it needs to find a way out. That way out is the toxic-lymphatic reaction.

At the spiritual level the theme of the toxic stage is 'movement'. Life itself wants to move stuck patterns and wants frozen structures to become dynamic, it wants to create transformation. It demands change, progress, evolution and needs continuous movement instead of stagnation.

THE BASIC TOXIC TREATMENT

Indication: all aggressive sicknesses with inflammations, chronic or regular colds especially in children, infections. This treatment activates the lymph flow, stimulates the elimination of waste products, helps to relieve pain.

It is important to observe the sequence of the points. Treat each point for 30 seconds. If unpleasant or negative reactions occur, stop treating that point and continue with the next one. The abbreviations for the acupuncture points are found in the annex.

Location of the points and sequence:

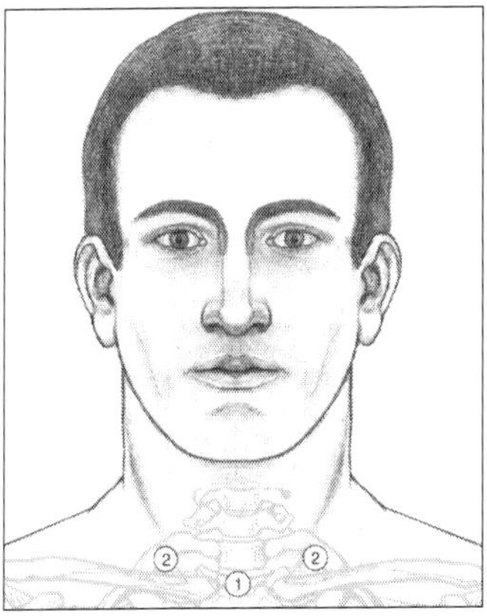

14 The basic toxic treatment – 1st step

1ST STEP

1 = CV 22, on the top edge of the sternum, in the hollow of the throat....................yellow

2 = Lymph 11, about 2 FW to the left and right of point 1, in the corner between the collarbone and the muscle that is clearly visible when you turn your head ....yellow

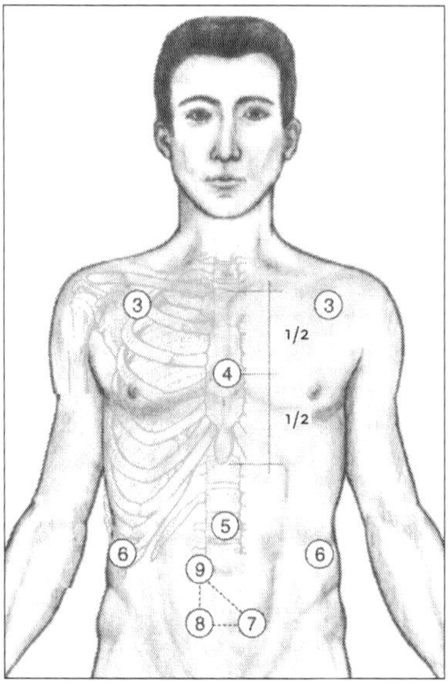

15 *The basic toxic treatment – 2nd step*

2ND STEP

3 = The drainage points of the lymph, near LU 1 under the collarbone, about 6 FW to the side of the middle line of the body .... yellow

4 = Peter Mandel calls this the 4th life stream point, in the middle of the sternum .... violet

5 = CV 12, on the middle line, exactly between the navel and the tip of the sternum (xyphoid) .... yellow

6 = LV 13, on the free tip of the 11th rib .... yellow

7-9 = The aggressive zones .... green

Location: these points or zones lie in a square, 2 FW from the middle of the navel, diagonally up, down, left and right. We only treat three points: first the one down on the left, then the point down on the right and finally the point up on the right.

These aggressive zones, that are located around the navel, form the lymph triangle that stimulates the lymph flow in the belly. By treating these zones we regulate the functioning of the small and large intestine and stimulate the elimination of waste products.

Peter Mandel calls them the aggressive zones, because the accumulation of waste products can become an aggressive element and turn against us. By radiating these points with green light we support the immune system that protects us against attacks from inside and outside.

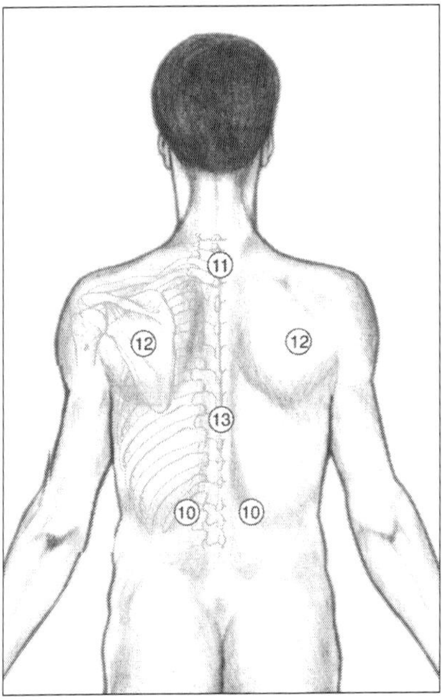

16 The basic toxic treatment – 3rd step

3RD STEP

10 = Kidney poles: they lie in the angle formed by the top lumbar vertebra L1 and the 12th rib ....red
11 = GV 14, under the protuberance of the 7th cervical vertebra...yellow
12 = SI 11, in the center of the shoulder blade, 1 FW up from the line that connects the armpits..........................yellow
13 = GV 9, under the protuberance of the 7th thoracic vertebra...yellow

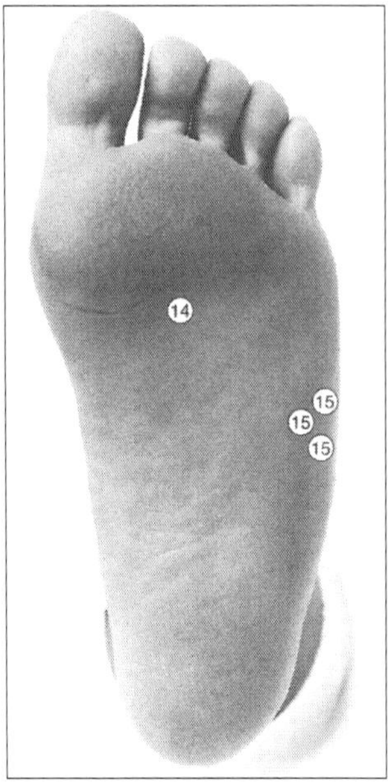

17 The basic toxic treatment – 4th step

14 = KD 1, on the sole of the foot between the metatarsal of the 2nd and 3rd toe (when bending the toes you find a hollow area) ....complementary green/red
15 = This is the area of the spleen in foot reflexology (only on the left foot) ....yellow or violet

If this area is sensitive to touch use violet, if not yellow. If you use the flat focus light set, you place the colored cap on this zone. If you use the light set for point treatment you test the area and treat the three most sensitive points in this area.

The degenerative stage

The third stage is called the degenerative stage. To describe it Peter Mandel uses terms such as rigidity, stagnation, immobility, the loss of living dynamics.

In regular medicine degenerative means that there are irreversible changes on the cellular level and in the bodily systems. Examples of degenerative diseases are rheumatism, arthritis, diabetics, cancer, multiple sclerosis. For Peter Mandel (and other naturopaths) much is still reversible, meaning that a disease could possibly be healed, either completely or partially. The condition for that to happen is that we take the road back from degeneration to regeneration, that there is a willingness to investigate negative patterns in behavior and mind-set.

At the spiritual level the degenerative stage indicates that life cannot develop any further, because there are emotional patterns and internal conflicts that this person cannot solve on his own. Help is needed from the outside.

With the next treatment we aim to stimulate the body in the degenerative stage to 'come back to life'. We try to instigate a reaction in order to break through stuck patterns. I elaborate more on degenerative diseases and their treatment in the final chapter of this book.

The basic degenerative treatment

First of all a disclaimer. Colorpuncture is not a substitute for a thorough medical diagnosis or treatment. Always consult your medical practitioner first if you have a serious complaint.

When the medical practitioner gives the diagnosis 'degenerative disease', it is certainly advisable to use the following treatment. Any degenerative disease can be treated with this sequence of eleven points. It is a general treatment that aims at starting the healing process – irrespective of the particular disease.

If you yourself have a degenerative disease – or someone in your family or circle of friends does – I do advise you to consult a colorpuncture therapist, acupuncturist or naturopath in your neighborhood. They can help you with a treatment plan and advise you on which treatments you can give at home.

You can also use the degenerative treatment if you feel stuck in life or in case other treatments don't bring proper results.

It is important to observe the sequence of the points. Treat each point for 30 seconds. If unpleasant or negative reactions occur, stop treating that point and continue with the next one. The abbreviations for the acupuncture points are found in the annex.

Location of the points and sequence:

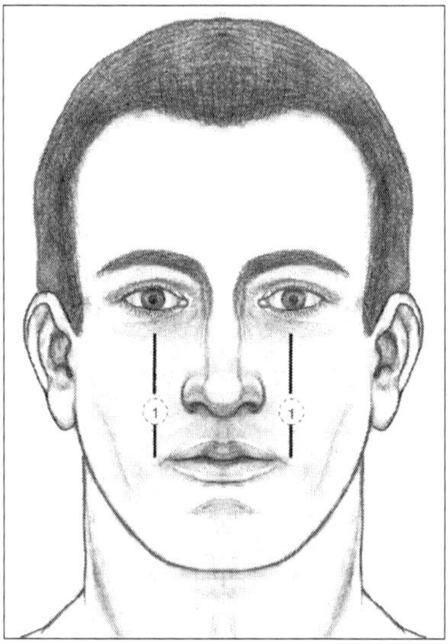

18 The basic degenerative treatment – 1st step

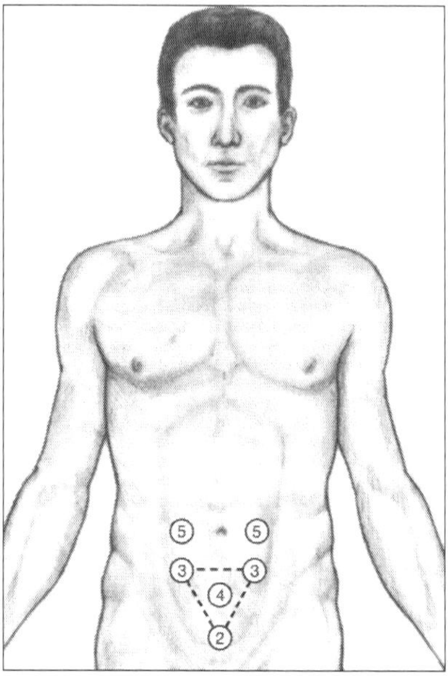

19 The basic degenerative treatment – 2nd step

1ST STEP

1 = Points of the facial cavities ....red
Location: at the lower edge of the cheekbone, straight below the pupils.

2ND STEP

2 = CV 3, about 2 FW up from the edge of the pubic bone, on the middle line ....red

3 = ST 27, 2 FW to the left and the right of the navel and 4 FW below it. First left, then right..red

4 = The center of the triangle CV3 and both points ST 27..........red

5 = ST 25, 2 FW left and right of the navel
....complementary yellow/violet
The more sensitive point gets violet, then the less sensitive point on the other side is treated with yellow.

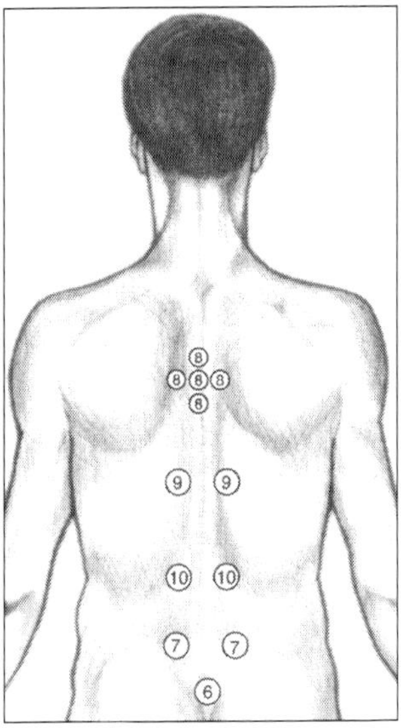

20 *The basic degenerative treatment – 3rd step*

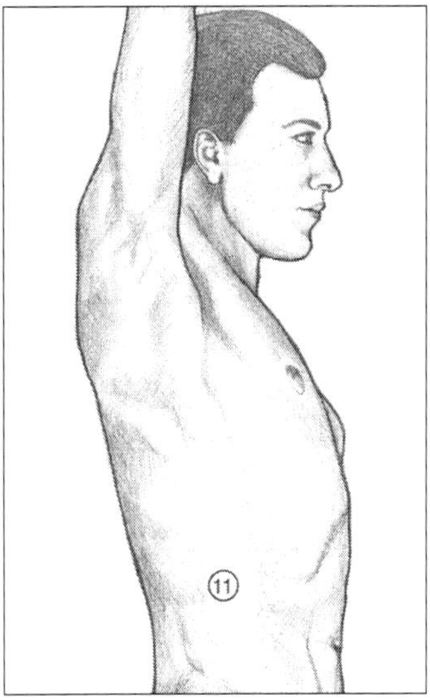

21 *The basic degenerative treatment – 4th step*

3RD STEP

6 = GV 2, at the top of the anal cleft..red

7 = UB 31, left and right, in the upper holes of the sacrum, 2 FW from the middle line..red

8 = Life cross or regeneration cross..red
The central point of this cross lies 1 FW above the middle of the horizontal line that connects both armpits. Peter Mandel calls this point the 3rd life stream point. The outer points of the cross lie at 1 FW from the center. Sequence of treatment: center, up, right, down, left.

9 = UB 18, next to the protuberance of the 9th thoracic vertebra, 2 FW from the middle of the spine ....complementary yellow/violet

10 = UB 23, treat complementary..................................red/green
UB 23: between L2 and L3 (lumbar vertebra 2 and 3), 2 FW from the middle of the spine.

4TH STEP

11 = GB 25, at the tip of the 12th rib
....complementary red/green

It is also possible to just massage the points or rub esogetic herbal oil on them. If you treat with light and color once or twice a week is sufficient. It helps to mitigate the complaints, it stimulates the body to become active and break through the stagnation. This treatment can also be given alongside medical treatments or if medication is taken that is prescribed by the physician. If you don't treat with colorpuncture, the esogetic herbal oil is best applied in the evening.

The color-sound therapy that is helpful in the degenerative stage of a sickness is the series Conflict Resolution (read more in chapter 10) and the series Totality: Body – Soul – Spirit.

Here is an example of how a sickness can develop from the endocrine via the toxic to the degenerative stage.

> *John experienced a lot of fear as a child. In his family he did not feel a sense of security, and the same was the case in school, among his friends. His mother and grandmother were also quite fearful, it seemed to run in the family. This fear influences the hormones (the adrenal glands – fight or flight) and belongs to the 'water' element in traditional Chinese medicine. The water element rules the bladder and the kidneys. In the endocrine stage fear is the main factor. Boys are often told: 'Big boys are not afraid.' They cannot express their fear and will quite likely repress it. As an adult John doesn't even know how it feels to be afraid. Maybe he wouldn't even recognize the feeling. After many years he gets a pyelitis. The toxic stage has arrived. More years pass and he needs an operation to remove kidney stones. That is the degenerative stage.*

This example shows that there is a connection between fear and kidney complaints. Other possible connections between emotions and organs are:

- Liver – dealing with anger. Also: flexibility, elasticity, assertiveness
- Lungs – sadness. Also: freedom, liberty
- Spleen and pancreas – worry and anxiety, loneliness. Also: being able to love yourself
- Large intestine – sadness. Also: the ability to let go
- Skin – difficulty to make contact. Also: to assert and guard your boundaries

5

Inner balance and well-being

We all feel tired or listless at times. There are daily conflicts at work or in the family. Sometimes our hormonal balance is disturbed and also mentally or emotionally we can be out of sync.

We experience a certain level of stress every day, which is not necessarily threatening for our health. But if stress accumulates and doesn't get released, it can have a negative influence on our well-being. Excessive stress levels or conflicts can lead to complaints varying from insomnia or a slight cold to a serious burnout or depression.

The following treatments can help you to regain your balance before any complaints start and to avert sickness. Prevention is better than cure. The treatments are easy to give and don't take much time. You can do them whenever you feel the need for them. They in fact give the informational and energetic system an overhaul, regulate the coordination between the brain hemispheres and have a positive effect on the hormonal balance.

Coordination 1 and 2

These two treatments form a pair. They help to harmonize the brain hemispheres.

Coordination 1 is best done in the morning and coordination 2 in the evening of the next day. You can continue this sequence of coordination 1 and 2 for a week or even longer. Such a treatment only takes five minutes, but the effect is immediate. They can also be combined with other treatments described in this book.

Coordination 2 works on other parts of the brain than coordination 1 and promotes a good rhythm of sleep. It is best to give this in the evening before going to sleep.

Coordination 1

Location of the points and sequence of treatment:

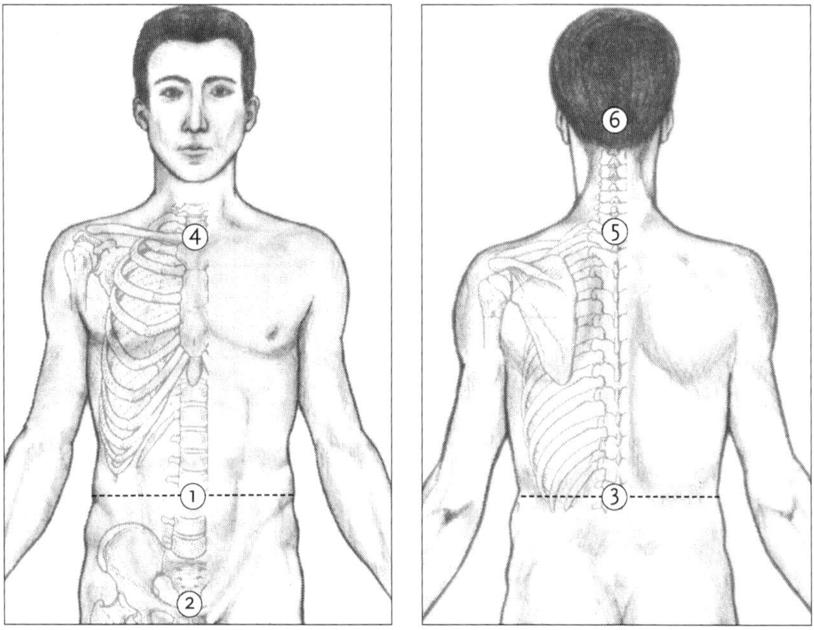

22 *Coordination 1*

1 = CV 8, the navel .... green
2 = CV 3, about 2 FW above the pubic bone, on the middle line .... orange
3 = On the back, on the spine, at the level of the navel .... violet
4 = CV 22, just under the throat, on the upper edge of the sternum in the hollow of the throat .... yellow
5 = GV 14, under the protuberance of the 7th cervical vertebra. When you feel along your neck, you find this cervical vertebra that sticks out a bit....... red
6 = GV 16, at the back of the head, in the hollow between the skull and the first cervical vertebra....... blue

All points are treated 30 seconds.

COORDINATION 2

Location of the points and sequence of treatment:

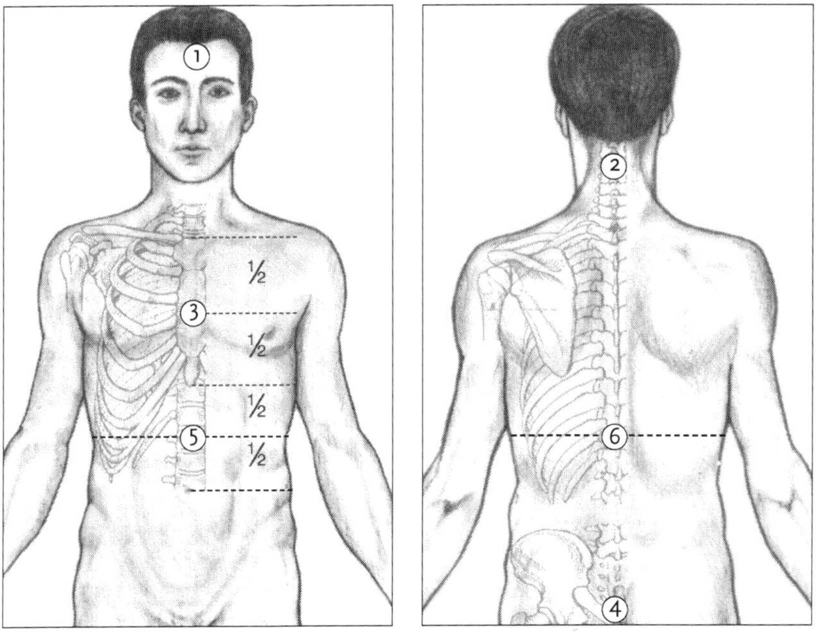

23 Coordination 2

1 = On the middle of the forehead, 1 FW under the hairline .... orange
2 = Between C4 en C5........ blue
Put your index finger on your neck and bend your head backwards. The point is located exactly in this fold on the spine.
3 = CV 17/18, in the middle of the sternum, right between the top and the lower tip of the sternum .... green
4 = GV 2: at the top of the anal cleft, where the coccyx starts........ red
5 = CV 12: between the navel and the tip of the sternum ......yellow
6 = On the back, on the spine opposite point 5 ....violet

All points are treated 30 seconds

Peter Mandel calls point 6 the point of life. It is one of the main points in colorpuncture. By treating this point you give the whole body a boost. Life energy starts to flow again.

The sound therapy that works best to restore your inner balance is the CD Psychosomatic Balance. It complements this treatment. In the annex you find more information on sound therapy.

If you have trouble getting started in the morning the red glasses can give you just that bit of extra strength that you need. Put them on for ten minutes and you will feel the effect.

Coordination crosses yin en yang

This treatment restores the balance between feeling and thinking. The left hemisphere of the brain is the seat of the rational, logical mind. The right hemisphere is the seat of feeling, spontaneity, creativity and intuition. Often these two hemispheres are not in balance. We call that a laterality disturbance.

This treatment helps to balance the two sides of the brain. You can give it to children who have difficulty to concentrate or suffer from ADHD – it is very helpful for them. See also chapter 8, in which I describe a few treatments especially suited for children.

Our life is dominated by polar opposites: day and night, warm and cold, male and female, life and death, positive and negative, active and passive, yin and yang, yes and no, thinking and feeling, for and against. When we are dominated by one pole or choose an extreme, we are in danger of losing our balance. As soon as we are balanced again, we can regard both poles as necessary complements.

Our life can be compared to that of a tight rope walker, who continuously has to balance to stay centered.

This treatment is helpful to find our balance and our centering.

Coordination crosses yin and yang

Location of the points:
Center of the cross in front: CV 12, between the navel and the tip of the sternum
Center of the cross in the back: the point opposite CV 12

Sequence of treatment and colors:

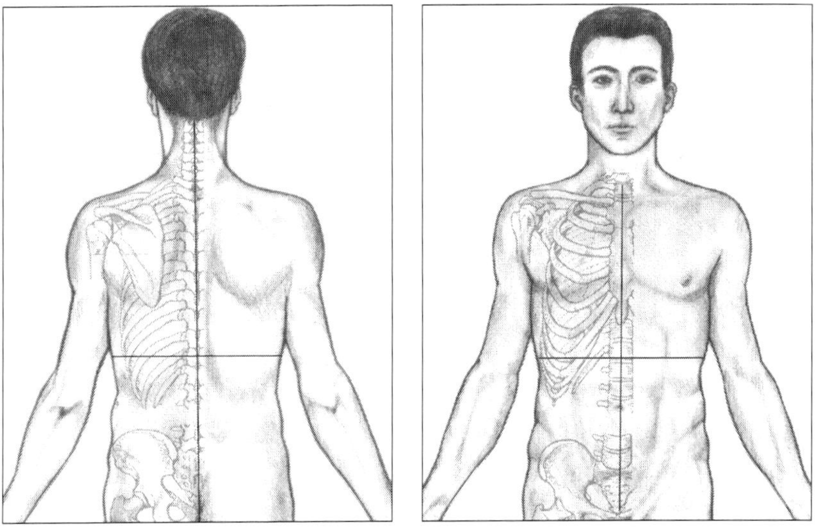

24 Coordination crosses yin and yang

Back:
Stroke the vertical line, starting up and going down, then up again, 4 – 5 times .... violet
Stroke the horizontal line from left to right and back, 4 – 5 times .... yellow

Front:
Stroke the vertical line, starting up and going down, then up again, 4 – 5 times .... yellow
Stroke the horizontal line from left to right and back, 4 – 5 times .... violet

Suitable sound therapy: CD Psychosomatic Balance

Coordination 10

This is a general treatment to help you if you feel too much pressure in the head.

COORDINATION 10

Location of the points and sequence of treatment:

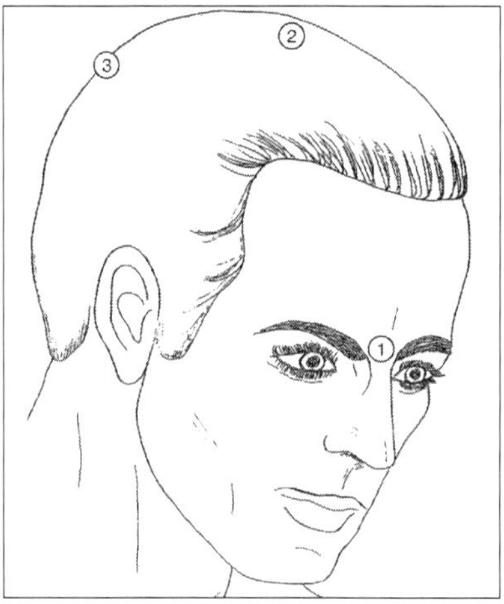

25 Coordination 10

1 = Yin trang ....blue
....(or violet, or orange)
Yin trang lies between the eyebrows.

2 = GV 20..blue
....(or violet, or orange)
GV 20: on the top of the head, in the middle (on the cross of the horizontal and vertical middle lines). Draw an imaginary line across the top of the head between the tips of the ears, the point is located on the middle line of the body.

3 = GV 19 ....blue
....(or violet, or orange)
GV 19: the point at the back of the head, where the skull curves down. About 4 FW behind GV 20 on the middle line.

This treatment can be done with three different colors. Not on the same day – choose one color and use it for a few days. You can use blue, orange or violet. These colors have different effects and indications.

- Blue: treat the three points with blue to treat sleeping disorders, pressure in the head, tensions, restlessness.

- Violet: treat the three point with violet in case of a trauma. This can be a physical trauma on the head, as caused by a fall or a concussion, but also disorientation or emotional pressure caused by any kind of trauma, even if it has taken place long ago.

- Orange: treat the three points with orange if you feel tired when you get up in the morning, or in case you feel depressed or have complaints due to menopause.

Treatment of body, soul and spirit on fingers and toes

Peter Mandel has been using kirlian photography for many years. A special camera takes a photo of fingertips and toes, which shows the weak radiation of light that the body emits in the form of a halo around each fingertip and toe. His knowledge of the meridians, almost all of which start or end in the fingers and toes, and his study of the kirlian photos taken of his patients over the years, enabled Peter Mandel to construct an interpretation model. The photos indicate where the complaints are located and to which organs they are related. In this book we shall not delve too deeply into this subject. On our website www.kleurenpunctuur.nl or www.esogetics.com you can find more information on kirlian photography. The interpretation of the kirlian photos have provided Peter Mandel with much information about the meaning associated with the fingers and toes, their relationship via the meridians to the organs and their interconnectedness.

In my own practice I use kirlian photography daily. If I notice, for instance, a slight deviation in the halo around the big toe, it indicates an energetic disturbance of the liver meridian or the spleen-pancreas meridian that starts there. According to traditional Chinese medicine the spleen represents the mind and complaints related to the head.

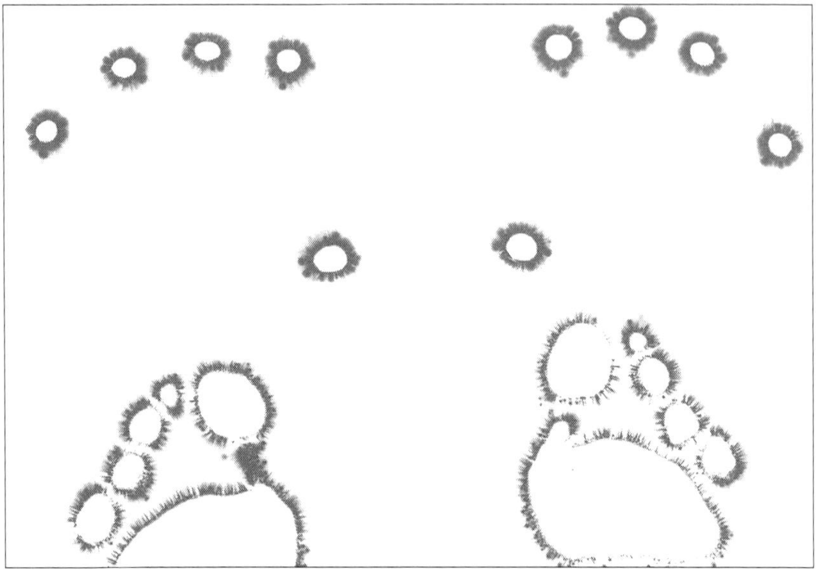

26 Kirlian photo

The toes are connected with the fingers, in accordance with the statement of Trismegistos 'as above, so below'. If I find certain deviations in the halo around the big toes and the thumbs, the interpretation model of Peter Mandel gives me the right starting point to treat the stagnant energy and help it to start flowing again. In the table you can find the meaning of the finger or toe which is most sensitive in your body.

Peter Mandel also assigned one of the ten classic planet symbols to each of our ten fingers. The fingers and toes are interrelated: the thumb is related to the big toe, the index finger to the second toe and so on. The sensitivity to pressure of the pads of fingers and toes can provide information about the background of certain complaints. Each finger or toe is connected to one or two classic acupuncture meridians and thereby to an organ or body system.

According to Mandel we can also find a reflection of our life cycle in our fingers and toes. Information about the start of our life is stored in the left little finger. Our life history then progresses via the left ring finger, middle finger, index finger and left thumb to the fingers of the

Fingers/ toes	Connected to	Planet	Meridians	Significance
Left little finger	Spirit	Sun	Heart and small intestine	Vitality, the start of life, the prenatal time, breathing in, the 'program' we have received at birth
Left ring finger	Spirit	Moon	Triple warmer and psyche	Seat of the hormonal system. We call this the finger of the subconscious and unconscious, of the feeling. The process of discovering the sense of 'I' around the age of 3 and the emotional patterns connected with that
Left middle finger	Soul	Mercury	Circulation and vascular degeneration	Intellect, rhythm, speech. Events around the age 6 and emotional patterns developed around that age and the marks they have left
Left index finger	Body	Venus	Large intestine and nerve degeneration	Love, erotic feelings, beauty. Events and conditionings around the age of 9
Left thumb	Body	Mars	Lungs and lymph	Energy, will, fighting spirit. Start of puberty around the age of 12
Right thumb	Body	Jupiter	Lungs and lymph	Abundance, wisdom, completion of the three phases of puberty: physically (around the age of 16), emotionally (around the age of 18) and spiritually (around the age of 25)
Right index finger	Body	Saturn	Large intestine and nerve degeneration	Limitation, hesitation
Right middle finger	Soul	Uranus	Circulation and vascular degeneration	Revolution, change, transformation
Right ring finger	Spirit	Neptune	Triple warmer and psyche	Deception, illusion, disintegration, sacrifice
Right little finger	Spirit	Pluto	Heart and small intestine	Collectivity, strength, power, a strong or weak ego, breathing out, death

right hand up to the right little finger. We then proceed to the small toe on the right foot and follow all toes until we reach the left small toe, which symbolizes the end of our life. Peter Mandel says all our fingers and toes represent a certain stage in life, where lessons have to be learned. In each finger or toe we meet our strong and our weak sides. A weak side can be with us from birth in order to learn a lesson. We can call these weak and strong aspects our karma, all factors that together constitute the lessons we need to learn in life.

In the table you find the meaning Peter Mandel assigns to the fingers. The toes are the 'reflection' of the fingers, as I have mentioned in chapter 2.

The next treatment aims at confirming our strengths and eliminating our weaknesses.

Coordination 8

This treatment of the pads of fingers and toes stimulates the general feeling of harmony, helps to dissolve blockages and strengthens the flow of information.

It is possible to treat all fingers and toes, or only the fingers or only the toes.

Apply the colored light to the pads of the fingers as described below. Start with the thumb of the left hand, continue along all fingers up to the little finger and then continue, starting with the thumb of the right hand up to the little finger. Treat each finger for 30 seconds. An unpleasant sensation during the treatment could point to the theme of that particular finger. Possibly some old, hidden conflicts start to dissolve. If you experience an unpleasant sensation, you switch to the complementary color for that finger.

Complementary colors:

Yellow – violet
Orange – blue
Red – green

Turquoise does not have a complementary color. If you experience an unpleasant feeling while treating the middle finger with turquoise, you stop and start treating the ring finger.

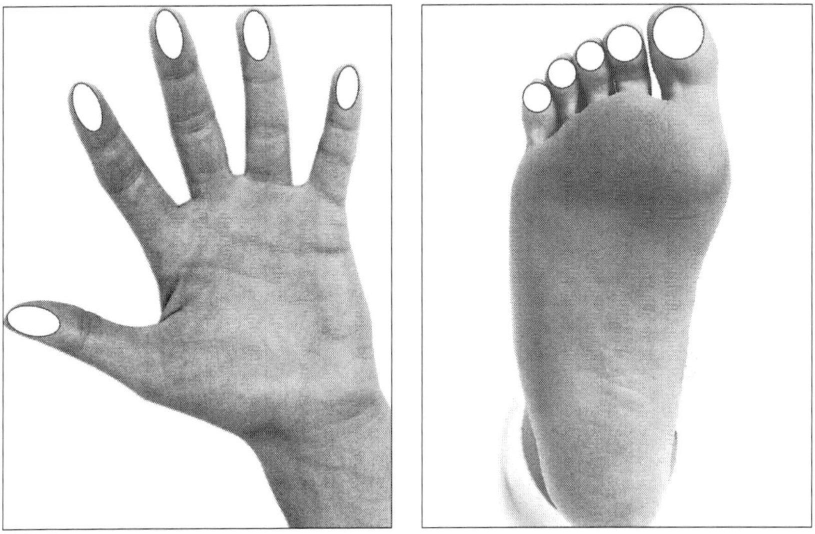

27 Coordination 8

You first treat the left hand and then the right hand using the following colors:
Thumb .... yellow
Index finger .... red
Middle finger .... turquoise
Ring finger .... blue
Little finger .... orange

Then you can start treating the toes. Start with the big toe on the left foot and continue till the small toe. Do the same on the right foot, again starting with the big toe.

The colors for the toes are:
Big toe .... orange
Second toe .... red
Middle toe .... turquoise
Fourth toe .... yellow
Small toe .... blue

If you experience an unpleasant reaction you switch to the complementary color for that toe. If this happens while you treat the middle toe with turquoise, you stop and continue with the next toe.

Over the last years I often taught a course called 'Light on the Foot' – a course especially designed for foot reflexology therapists. Many of them apply this treatment on the toes of their clients and I often hear the remark that this helps their clients to relax in a way they have not experienced before. Massaging the feet afterwards is so much easier and goes deeper.

The sound therapy series Totality: Body – Soul – Spirit supports this treatment and helps you regain your balance.

6

Headache and migraine

Headaches are tricky, not just for the person suffering from them, but also for the therapist. The causes can be many and are often hard to diagnose. Specialized headache clinics exist, where medical staff do countless tests in order to arrive at a diagnosis and to find a suitable treatment. In Chinese medicine more than a hundred types of headache are described. That shows how much patience both the therapist and the client require in order to investigate the cause of the complaints. An easy way out is to take a painkiller, but that is a temporary solution that does not solve the problem. It is always important to figure out the reason why this occurs. Not acting, or just fighting the symptoms, leads to a cul-de-sac and can do a lot of damage. It is always advisable to have a thorough medical examination first to get an indication of possible causes.

Most people suffering from migraines don't quite know what triggers it. In his clinic Peter Mandel discovered that the cause of a headache can often be found in the area of the stomach and the intestines. In that case there are accompanying complaints such as diarrhea, constipation or acidity of the stomach. A malfunctioning liver or gallbladder can also lead to cramps in the veins of the head. If that is the case, you can find some treatments in chapter 9 that can be combined with the treatments in this chapter.

Another form of headache is the cervicogenic headache, which starts with pain at the back of the head and is often accompanied by simultaneous eye pressure, disturbance of equilibrium, vein cramps and light flashes in the eyes. In this case the cause may be a slipped disk in the cervical vertebrae. Because the meridians of the gallbladder and the bladder run through the neck, the complaint could be related to these organs.

Infections in the molars or the jaw and amalgam fillings can also cause a headache.

Another type of headache is related to eye complaints or pressure on the eyes. New reading glasses can offer a solution in some cases. In Chinese medicine, and also in esogetic holistic medicin, the eyes are related to the liver energy. The liver is connected with strong emotions, as explained in chapter 9. Strong emotional stress, that has not been processed, can be the cause. Spending too much time at the computer can also lead to headache. These are just a few examples.

And what is a migraine? A real migraine comes in attacks. It is a one-sided headache, which can last for hours or even days. Possible causes are:

- medication;
- sensitivity to certain weather patterns, such as low atmospheric pressure or snow;
- certain herbs or spices that lead to an allergic reaction;
- stimulants such as alcohol. We all know the hangover after excessive drinking that brings on a headache. Sometimes the coloring agent in red wine is the culprit, not the alcohol. Also chocolate, licorice or artificial food additives can cause an allergic reaction that results in a headache;
- hormonal disturbances or menstrual disorders women often have.

In my practice I always start by making a kirlian photo of fingers and toes. This gives me an indication which organs and meridians are related to the complaint. I also inquire extensively into the life history of the client in order to get an overview of the total syndrome. It can also be useful for the client to keep a 'headache diary' and note down in which situation the headache occurs.

> *Nancy came to my practice because of her migraine. Every four weeks she had a serious attack with nausea and vomiting. The attack always occurred on the day before her menstruation started. My assumption was that I needed to regulate her hormonal balance. I gave her some endocrine treatments, but they didn't help her. During her next visits I asked her some more questions and it turned out that a day before her menstruation started she felt a craving for licorice. She bought a big bag of a certain brand and gobbled it all up. It gave her some consolation, as she felt melancholic. The licorice helped her, she told me. I asked her just for once not to eat*

the licorice. That month she didn't get a headache. She experimented with it and discovered she was allergic to licorice. After she stopped eating licorice, her headaches disappeared.

Here are some treatments that you can give yourself. Try them out and after some time you will know which one works best for you.

COORDINATION 10

Indication: sleeping disorders, headache caused by tension, restlessness.

Location of the points and sequence of treatment:

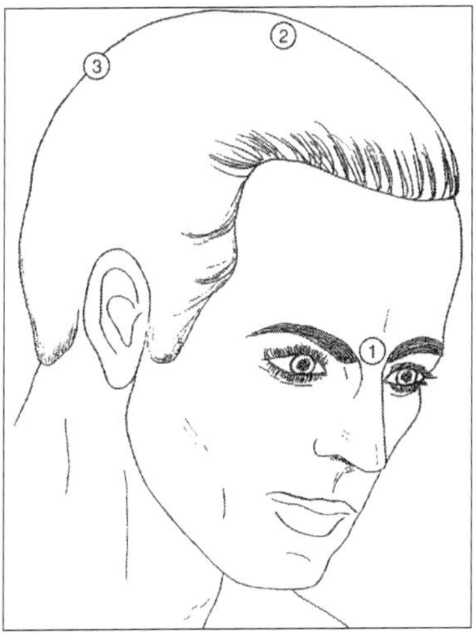

28 *Coordination 10*

1 = Yin trang .... blue (or violet)
Yin trang: between the eyebrows on the middle line.
2 = GV 20 .... blue (or violet)
GV 20: on the top of the head, in the middle, at the cross point of the horizontal and vertical line.
3 = GV 19 .... blue (or violet)
GV 19: the point at the back of the head where the skull curves down. About 4 FW behind GV 20 on the middle line.

Treat all three points with blue to calm down mental activity. Use violet if you are dealing with a lot of emotional tension.

All points are treated 30 seconds.

BASIC MIGRAINE TREATMENT

Here we treat the so-called life stream points. The explanation about the life streams according to Peter Mandel is found in chapter 7.

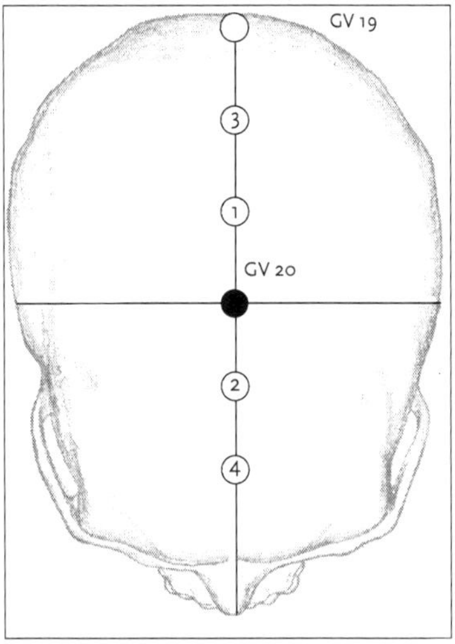

29 1st step: Migraine

1ST STEP: LIFE STREAM POINTS ON THE SKULL

1 = ...red
2 = ...green
3 = ...yellow
4 = ...blue

The points all lie on the vertical middle line of the skull. Divide the line between GV 20 and the hairline in three equal sections. The points 2 and 4 are located at 1/3 and 2/3 of the distance to GV 20.

Also divide the line between GV 20 and GV 19 in three equal sections. Point 1 is located at 1/3 behind GV 20 and point 3 at 2/3 behind GV 20.

GV 20 lies on the top of the skull, on the middle line. GV 19 lies 4 FW behind GV 20 on the middle line, where the skull curves down.

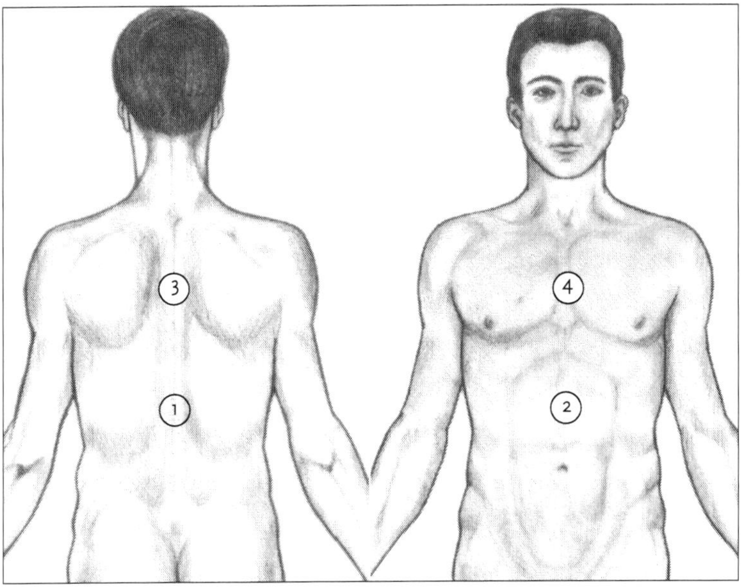

30 2nd step: Migraine

2ND STEP: LIFE STREAM POINTS ON THE BODY

1 = Opposite CV 12 on the spine..red
2 = CV 12..green
3 = 1 FW above the line connecting the armpits, on the spine...yellow
4 = CV 17/18: in the middle of the sternum..............................blue

Location of the points:
Locate point 2 first, this is the acupuncture point CV 12 and lies on the middle line between the navel and the tip of the sternum. Draw an imaginary horizontal line from CV 12 to the back. On that horizontal line, on the spine, lies point 1, opposite point 2. Point 3 is located on the spine, 1 FW up from a horizontal line connecting both armpits. Point 4 lies opposite point 3, in the middle of the sternum.

Treat the life stream points in the sequence 1-4. First massage them and then treat them with colored light, 30 seconds each.

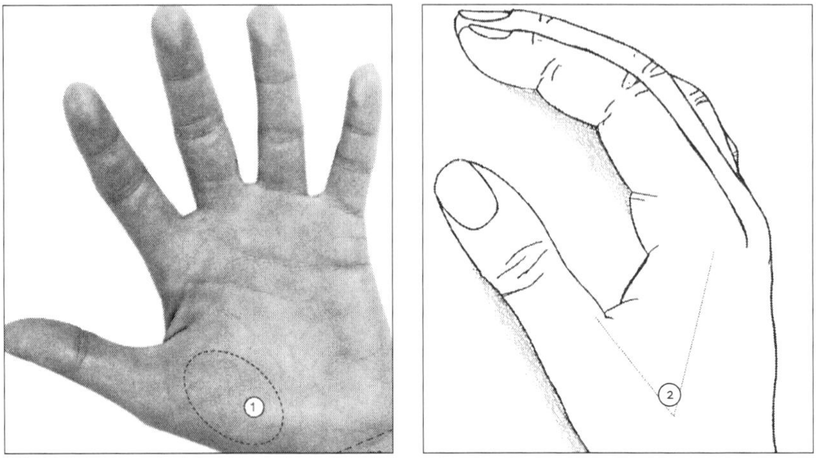

31 3rd step: Migraine points on the hand

3RD STEP: MIGRAINE POINTS ON THE HAND

1= The point for the head on the hand ....red
This point lies on the heel of the hand, under the thumb. The point is sensitive to pressure. Treat the point first on the left hand, then on the right hand.

2 = LI 4...blue
This point lies in the webbing between thumb and index finger and is always sensitive to pressure. Treat the point first on the left hand, then on the right hand. Don't treat this point if pregnant.

4TH STEP: NEURASTHENIA LINE ON THE FOREHEAD

The neurasthenia line is used in Chinese scalp acupuncture, where the line is treated with needles. Peter Mandel has discovered that stroking this line with violet light has an immediate effect in relaxing the mind and the head. If you find it difficult to fall asleep, treating this line is helpful if done just before going to bed. It also helps agitated children to calm down.

This line lies 1 FW up from yin trang, the point between the eyebrows. The outer points of the line are situated over the pupils of the eye, when looking straight ahead.

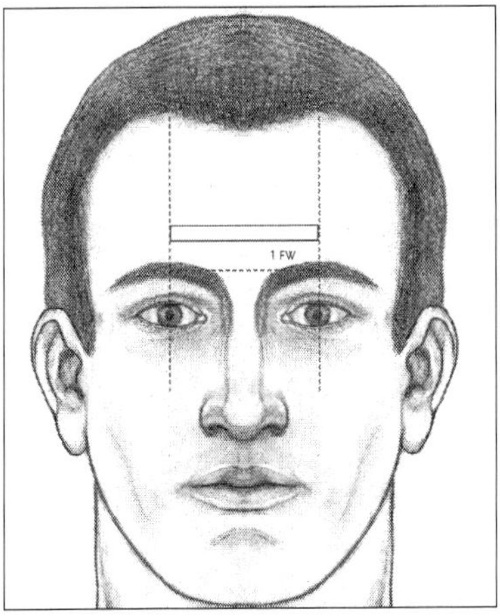

32 *4th step: Migraine – neurasthenia line*

Neurasthenia line ....violet
Stroke the line on the forehead slowly from the left to the right and back, 5 times.

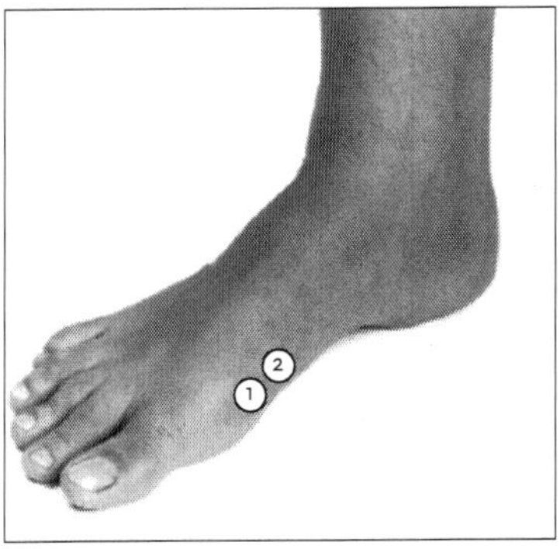

33 *5th step: Migraine – SP 4*

5TH STEP: ACUPUNCTURE POINT SP 4

SP 4: Treat complementary ....green/red
Finding SP 4 (point 2) is easy if you first locate SP 3 (point 1). SP 3 lies just behind the base joint of the big toe. SP 4 is found 2 FW behind SP 3.

Test SP 4 on the left and the right foot to find which point is most sensitive. The more sensitive point is treated first with the cool color green. Then the less sensitive point on the other foot is treated with red.

If you often suffer from a migraine and you feel the onset of an attack, it can be helpful to massage SP 4 vigorously for 10 minutes, left and right. In this way you can avoid the attack.

Listening to the CD Migraine/Headache can also give relief. Can also be combined with the CD Psychosomatic Balance, especially if the headache is related to the hormonal cycle.

Sometimes the solution is surprisingly easy, as the next example from my practice illustrates.

> *David came to my practice for treatment – headache was one of his complaints. He suffered from headaches almost daily and wanted to stop taking painkillers. During my first treatment I asked him to take off his glasses. When he did, I noticed the indents from the frame on the side of his face. He had put on quite a bit of weight over the years and the frame didn't fit any longer. I advised him to see an optician and get the frame adjusted. He cancelled his next appointment as he no longer had a headache.*

If the headache is connected to your menstrual cycle (e.g. it always comes on the second day of your period or on the day of ovulation), the endocrine treatment as described in chapter 4 is your best option.

Stress as a cause of headache

A headache is often caused by stress. We are strained, our head is overloaded and we are off balance. What is stress? It is not a sickness, but actually a natural and valuable defense mechanism of our body, that not only serves humankind, but is found everywhere in nature, also in plants and animals. Stress in itself is not harmful, even when it forces us to extreme exertion. It is only hazardous if the excessive energy mobilized by stress stays in our system and cannot be released. The burden then becomes permanent and without exception leads to sickness.

In his book *New Land of Thinking* Frederic Vester described this as follows:

'Stress prepares the body to climb trees, jump at the enemy with loud screaming or swim across a river. This happens through the release of three hormones: The flight hormones epinephrine, and the attack hormone norepinephrine, which both stimulate circulation and override thought in favor of preprogrammed reflex actions, as well as cortisol which increases blood coagulation, quiets digestive and sexual functions and suppresses the immune function – all in order to better focus on the fight and to create a better outcome.'

Nowadays it seems we are subconsciously preprogrammed to strive for more material possessions and to fight hard to achieve more and more in life. The stress this creates has become a health hazard and is now a permanent factor in our daily life. By wanting more all the time, we enter a vicious circle. We aren't capable of releasing the tensions and hardly know how it feels to be in peace and quiet. Children already learn at an early age in school that they have to perform in order to be appreciated.

Due to this unnatural development our cells, organs and our autonomic nervous system can be thrown off balance. The permanent presence of hormones such as epinephrine, norepinephrine and cortisol in the body indicates that the delicate balance between tension and relaxation is disturbed. This results in a latent burden on our entire body, which can be the starting point for potentially more serious diseases. If the two poles of stress and relaxation can be kept in balance, it is easier to live a healthy life and probably avoid a great number of diseases – especially all cardiovascular diseases, which are still the main cause of death in our hectic world. Stomach complaints. digestive and intestinal disorders, impotence, a weak immune system and failing powers of concentration are often caused by a buildup of stress. The rise in cancer in the past decades is often thought to be related to the permanent stress level and unsolved inner conflicts, even though there are many other possible causes, such as heredity, radiation and environmental pollution.

As soon as a sickness occurs, the first reaction usually is to treat the symptoms, often without finding or removing the root cause. Stomach aches are repressed by taking a pill. Medication is given to try to suppress excessive aggression. Fatigue, lethargy, neuroses e.g. are all fought with drugs and regular infections treated with antibiotics. It is easy to see that this leads to a vicious circle. The medication represses the symptoms, but the root cause is not eliminated. The sickness becomes chronic and in that stage heavier medication is needed to make life bearable, although healing may not be possible any more. Therefore Peter Mandel always insists that we search for the true root cause that lies hidden behind the symptomatic complaints. If these causes can be taken away or prevented, there is no need for us to get sick.

Brain waves and induction therapy

If you suffer from headaches regularly, it will be good to find ways to relax. Yoga, relaxation exercises or meditation can help to create a refuge for yourself. You need to learn how to release the buildup of tension again and again. Easier said than done – many people find it difficult to be in a state of deep relaxation or to find ways to release tension. Peter Mandel therefore researched brain waves to find out how they are connected to stress-related physical and emotional complaints.

Here is an overview of the main brain rhythms and their effect:

Beta rhythm
The beta rhythm is described as an irregular small wave with a frequency of 14 to 30 Hz. It represents the concentration directed to the outside world and an alert, awake state of being. Logical thinking, intellectual and intense mental activity are an expression of beta waves, also feelings of restlessness and a tendency to worry. A high number of beta waves leads to a high level of stress hormones, such as adrenaline and noradrenaline.

Alpha rhythm
Alpha waves have a frequency of 7.5 to 13.5 Hz and are typical for a state of relaxation and intellectual composure. They arise when we close our eyes and induce a feeling of pleasant rest. The alpha rhythm is present at the start of meditative relaxation, when body and mind are in a harmonious state.

Theta rhythm

Theta waves have a frequency of 4 to 7 Hz and belong to certain phases of sleep and deep meditation. Deep layers of consciousness are accessed. Intellectual mind processes are no longer functioning, but imagination, visionary memories, intuition and fantasy are fully active. In this wavelength the capacity to learn is at its peak, because the filter of analytical thought is not working. Maybe this is the reason why theta waves are prominent in children.

Delta rhythm

Delta waves – 0.5 to 3.5 Hz – have a very low frequency and are typical for deep, dreamless sleep. They are seldom found in the awake state. Delta frequencies are important for healing processes, for regeneration and a proper functioning of the immune system. Delta waves are a prerequisite for deep hypnosis and trance states.

Disturbances in the brain rhythm can lead to headache and also to the inability to attain deep relaxation. If we stay in the beta rhythm we may find it hard to change over to the other rhythms that are necessary for relaxing and going to sleep. Much research has been done over the years about brain rhythms, mainly with the aim to find possibilities to stimulate certain rhythms or to balance the different frequencies. Neurofeedback therapy is one of these new methods that uses brain waves.

For many years Peter Mandel also researched the relationship between disease and brain waves. He developed his own therapy, using induction of equal impulses in order to restore the natural state of the brain waves. Unlike neurofeedback he doesn't use auditory or visual stimuli, but impulses via the skin. In induction therapy weak electric impulses of a certain frequency enter the body via the skin. The same impulses are also found in the brain itself and can therefore be called equal impulses. In case of sickness the electric currents in the brain show a slight deviation. The impulses that are given stimulate the brain to switch to the right frequency and in this way can reduce complaints or even take them away. It is a safe and painless treatment that restores the balance between the brain waves. The appliance that transmits these impulses to the skin is called 'Synapsis home special' and is suited for home treatment. Peter Mandel has developed

26 different programs, aimed at better sleep, relaxation, improved learning (also for children), lowering stress levels. There are also programs for people suffering from depression. A selection of three of these programs can be downloaded on a Synapsis home special.

I used the program 'Rest 1' for many years. The treatment takes half an hour and afterwards I felt as if I had had a good night's sleep. Now it seems my brain can automatically switch to a state of relaxation and I don't need to use this program any more. Especially in stressful or busy times it can be very helpful to use such an induction program twice or thrice a week to learn to relax, to improve sleep or to cope with traumatic experiences.

7 Strengthening the immune system

In this chapter we focus on the immune system that protects us against attacks from bacteria and other pathogens. The main topic here is how we can strengthen our immune system and become less vulnerable to infections or colds. I don't discuss congenital defects of the immune system or auto-immune diseases in this context. I rather aim at giving a deeper understanding of the development of diseases and I offer some tips how to recognize the early warning signals.

A strong or a weak immune system is determined by a multitude of factors, such as environmental influences, nutrition, hereditary or genetic factors, stress at work or in relationships, radiation (also from electronic devices), a lack of fresh air and sunlight, intake of alcoholic beverages, smoking, drugs – it is a long list. In many of these areas you can boost your immune system by making the right choices in your daily life.

Some people have a strong immune system, others don't. One person may catch a cold at the slightest breeze, someone else can walk for hours in bad weather without being affected. When there is an epidemic flu, many people don't get sick, even though they may be in close contact with flu patients at home or in the medical profession. Some just don't catch the flu, even if they have not been given an influenza vaccination.

In esogetic holistic medicine fever, sinusitis or a sore throat are not regarded as a sickness, but as a natural and useful reaction of the immune system. Far too often antibiotics are prescribed, which disturb the natural process of healing. Nowadays the medical profession is more aware of the danger of immunity to antibiotics. Nevertheless, there is no doubt that we should be grateful for the help antibiotics provide in case of life threatening diseases.

The esogetic approach is always to try and strengthen the immune system and our defenses. We want to help the body to weather such a temporary crisis by itself, maybe aided by homeopathic or other natural remedies. The treatments aim at assisting the body to quickly discharge toxic waste via the kidneys, intestines, lungs and skin, because this is the natural way. If you observe a person who has a fever, you will notice that they want to drink a lot (which helps the discharge via the kidneys) and don't have an appetite for food (the intestines get a cleaning). The body seems to go on a natural fast. Sweating profusely helps to discharge toxic waste via the skin and by coughing phlegm is brought up from the lungs.

In this context Peter Mandel stresses the importance of the lymph system and I would like to give you some more information on it.

The importance of the lymph for the immune system

The three main lymph areas

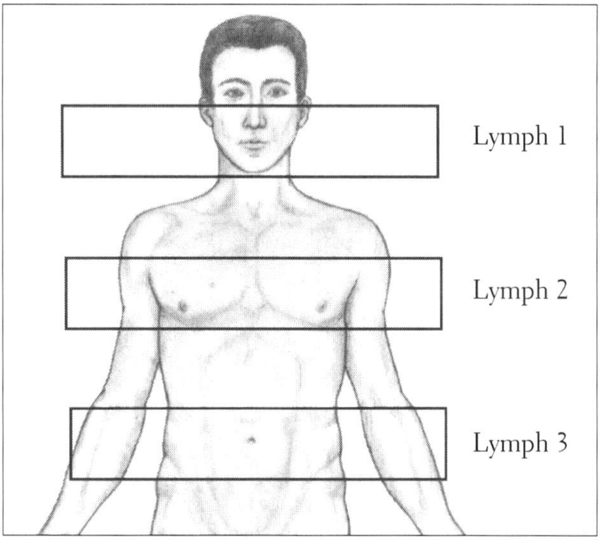

34 *The three main lymph areas*

According to Peter Mandel there are three main lymph areas – head, chest and lungs, and the belly. The head area serves as a pump, each breath activates the lymph flow. The discharge of waste partly takes place in the area of chest and lungs. The lymph area in the belly processes the remaining waste and supports the elimination. Peter Mandel calls these areas the focal resonance zones, because they are resonating among each other. If there is a disturbance in the lymph area of the head, such as a chronic sinusitis, a scar from a tonsillitis or an infection of the jaw, the other lymphatic areas are also affected.

Connection between the lymphatic system and the central nervous system

It is a well-known fact that the lymphatic system and the central nervous system are connected. We know that inflammation in the teeth or in the cavities can cause disturbances in the nerves of the brain or in the organs. It is less well-known that lymphatic disorders in childhood can be the cause of complaints, sickness or pain in adulthood. Examples are regular or chronic tonsillitis, ear infections, sinusitis, bronchitis or intestinal complaints in childhood. These infections can leave scars that play up as a focal inflammation. Therefore it is important to see the connection between patterns of disease in the past and the actual complaints.

Peter Mandel has discovered four zones on the top of the skull where memories of past diseases, such as an appendicitis, tonsillitis or operation, are apparently stored in the brain. One could say that an emotional scar is left behind that causes disturbances in the energy flow, which can lead to complaints like rheumatism, arthritis or spinal ailments. Treating these four zones often helps to release that old pain and the result is a deep state of relaxation and a feeling of relief.

THE LYMPH ZONES ON THE SKULL

On the top of the skull, exactly in the center, lies an circular area with a diameter of 2 finger widths. Therapists sometimes refer to it as a channel. Within this circle four important 'psychological buffer points' are found on the two diagonals, about half a finger width from the center. Experiences from childhood are stored here. You can massage this area vigorously with your fingers and rub three drops of esogetic herbal oil on it. This stimulates dream activity and will after some time lead to a feeling of inner liberation.

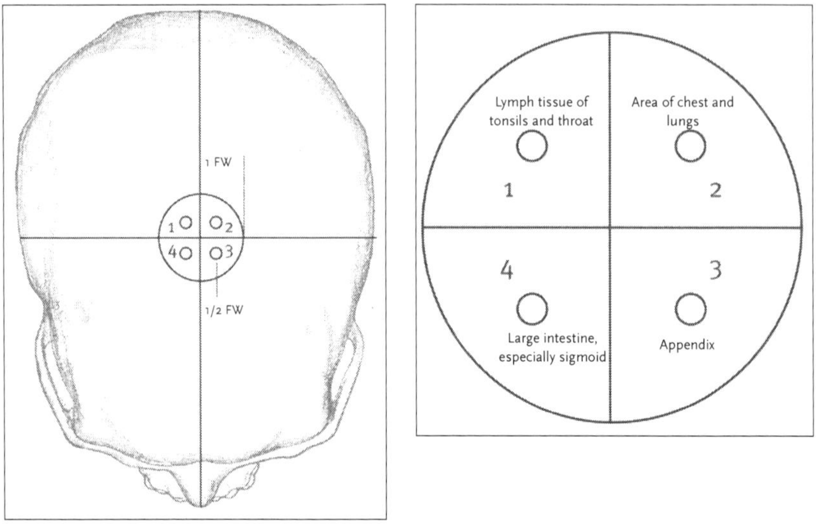

35 *The lymph zones on the skull*

1 = Point for lymph tissue of tonsils and throat
2 = The area of chest and lungs
3 = Appendix
4 = Large intestine, especially sigmoid colon

THE BASIC TOXIC TREATMENT

This is one of the main treatments that helps to strengthen the immune system and to activate the body's own defenses. It activates the flow of the lymph, stimulates the elimination of waste and alleviates pain. The description of this treatment can be found in chapter 4.

Other ways to eliminate toxins

A good way to detoxify your body is to take a footbath with esogetic herbal oil once or twice a week. Put ten drops of this oil in a basin filled with hot water (the temperature should be about 39° Celsius). Sit down and put your feet in the hot water for ten minutes and then rest them for fifteen minutes, wrapped in a warm towel.

There are several ways in which you can help yourself and your family members to have a better functioning lymph system. I already mentioned the basic toxic treatment that is suitable for everyone. Just massaging the points or rubbing them with esogetic herbal oil is also an option, best done at night.

If you use colorpuncture for the basic toxic treatment, once or twice a week is sufficient to strengthen the immune system. In many cases it can prevent the onset of a disease.

Listening to the CD Immune Activity is an additional support in treating all toxic complaints.

The yellow glasses also stimulate the activity of the lymph. The turquoise glasses are effective for all allergic complaints such as hay fever.

A general advice to help you improve your immune system is to move the body. Both medical and holistic natural healers agree that we need to be more active, we need to do physical exercise. When we move, our breathing becomes deeper, we give our muscles a work-out. They in turn activate the lymph system which eliminates the toxins.

You have probably experienced the uncluttered, healthy feeling you have after running, cycling or playing sports. Sweating has eliminated a lot of toxins, your lymph system has cleansed your body and suddenly you see solutions that you didn't see before.

Research has shown that it is better to do sports outdoors than indoors in a hall. You take in a good dose of sunlight for free!

General treatments for common complaints

Here are a few extra treatments for common complaints. They can be alternated with the basic toxic treatment that is described in chapter 4.

If you often suffer from one of these complaints, it would be good to check for yourself which events preceded an onset and how you have dealt with (emotional) stress.

COMMON COLD, FLU AND SINUSITIS

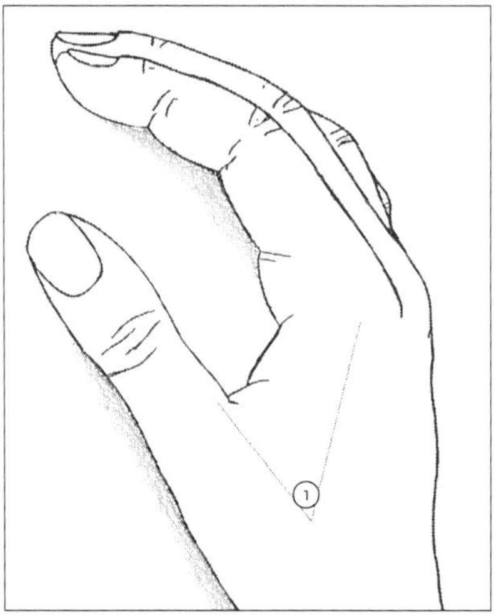

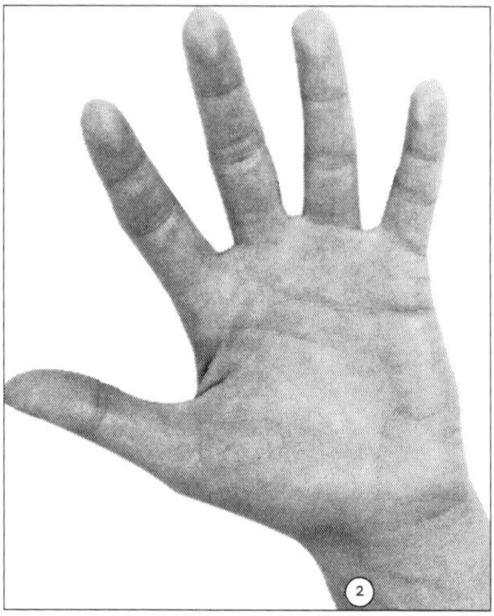

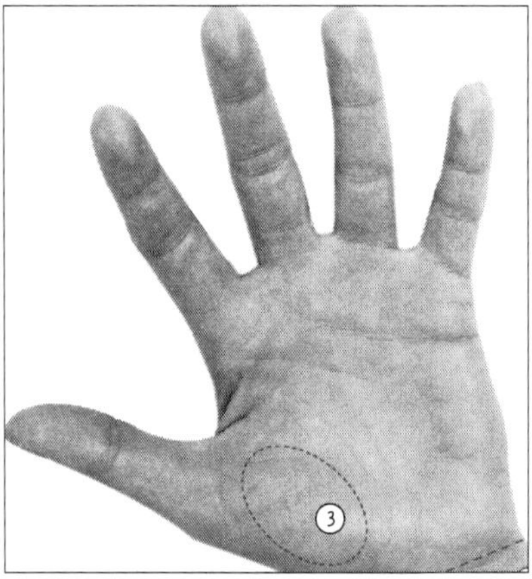

36 Common cold and sinusitis

1 = LI 4: on both hands in the webbing between thumb and index finger on top of the hand .... red
Don't treat this point if pregnant.
2 = LU 7: 2 FW under the first fold of the wrist .... red
3 = In the lower third of the heel of the hand .... red

All points are first treated on the left, then on the right, each point or zone about 30 seconds.

COMMON COLD, FLU AND SINUSITIS – EXTRA TREATMENT

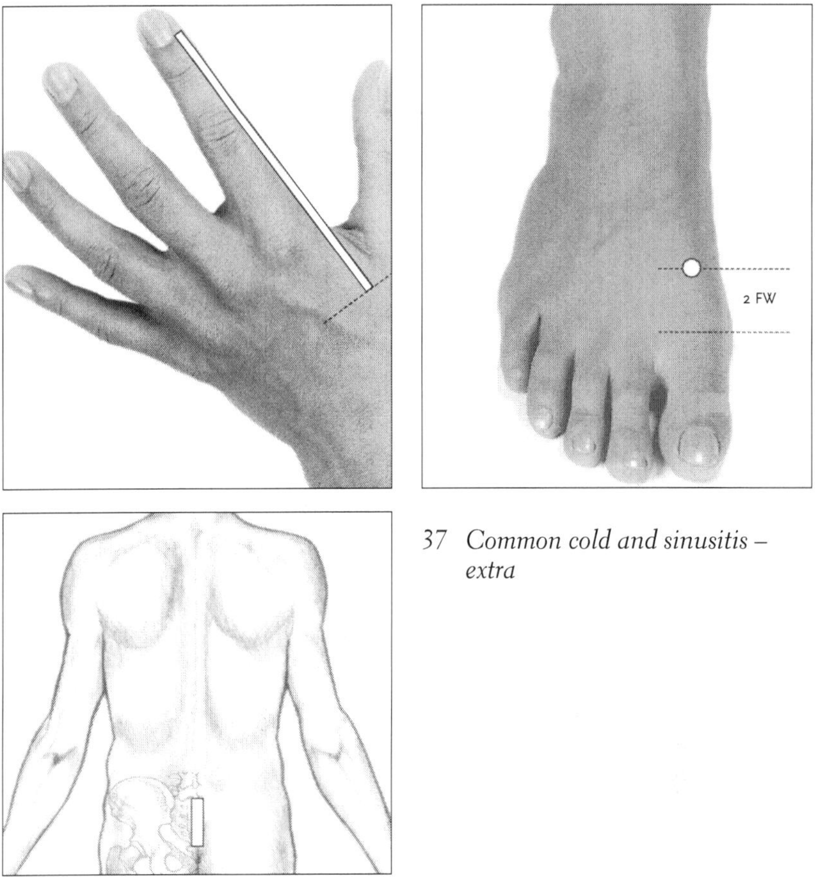

37 *Common cold and sinusitis – extra*

Line of the large intestine meridian on the index finger................red
Lymph zone on the foot..yellow or violet

If the zone is painful, use violet, otherwise yellow.
This zone is located halfway the arch of the foot, between the metatarsals of the big toe and the second toe.

Line on sacrum/pelvis ....red

Stroke the vertical line in the middle of the sacrum.
The top of this line lies on the 5th lumbar vertebra and the end on the beginning of the anal cleft. Stroke the line 5 times up and down.

SKIN RASHES AND ECZEMA

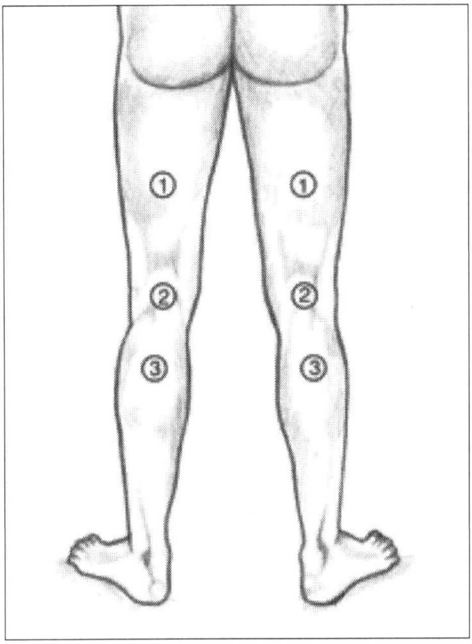

38 *Skin rashes and eczema*

1 = UB 37 ....red
UB 37: in the middle of the back of the thigh
2 = UB 40 ....red
UB 40: in the middle of the back of the knee
3 = 1 handbreadth below the hollow of the knee ....red

The back of the knee is notorious for skin rashes. If you acutely suffer from a rash, use green instead of red on point 2. The other points are treated with red, unless there is a rash there as well, in that case use green.

This treatment also works well for itches anywhere on the body. Also use red here, only if you have a skin rash on these points green should be used.

All points are treated left and right, each point or zone 30 seconds.

COUGH AND BRONCHITIS

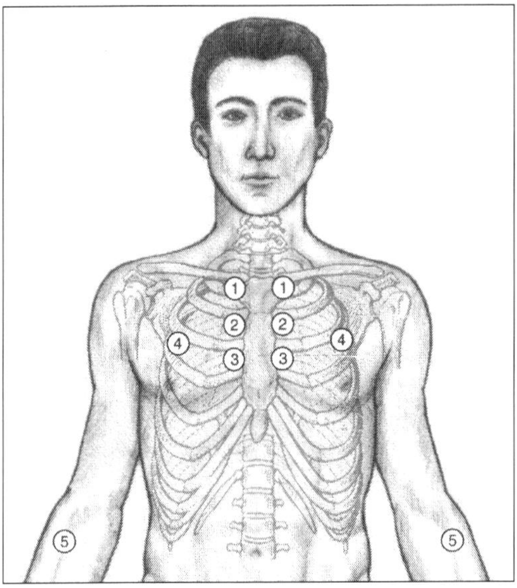

39 *Cough and bronchitis*

1 = KD 27, treat complementary .... green/red
2 = KD 26, treat complementary .... green/red
3 = KD 25, treat complementary .... green/red
4 = Converter points for the kidneys,
first left, then right .... green
5 = LU 5, treat complementary .... green/red

Points 1, 2 and 3 are located between the ribs, 2 FW from the sternum. Points 4 lie between the 3rd and 4th rib. Find the middle of the collarbone and go 4 FW down. Between the 3rd and the 4th rib you find a point that is sensitive to pressure – it is sensitive for everyone. These points regulate the lymph drainage from the head and are connected with the kidneys through the principle of the inverted man. I have explained this principle in chapter 2. Points 5 lie in the fold of the elbow, at the thumb side of the tendon that lies in the fold of the elbow.

Points 1, 2, 3, and 5 are treated complementary: test each point left and right. The more sensitive point is treated with the cool color green first, the less sensitive point is then treated with red.

Joints

The following treatment is good to apply if you have swollen and painful joints. It can be used on fingers, toes, knees, hips or shoulders.

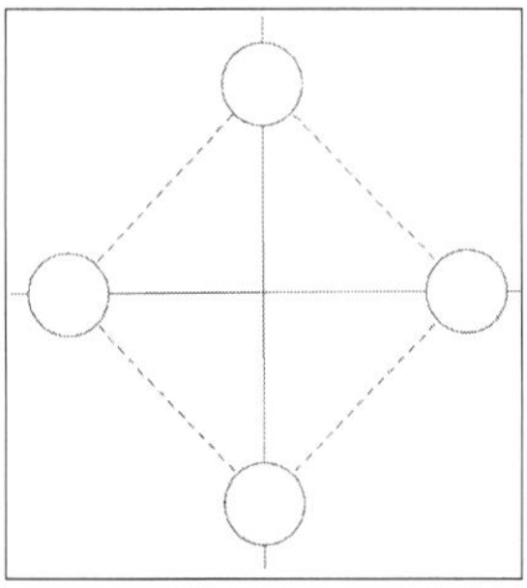

Esogetic principle of the joints: Around each joint there are four points in the form of a cross. Test the points for sensitivity. One of the points will be the most painful. Treat that point with green, the others with red.

Sequence: treat the red points first, then the green point.

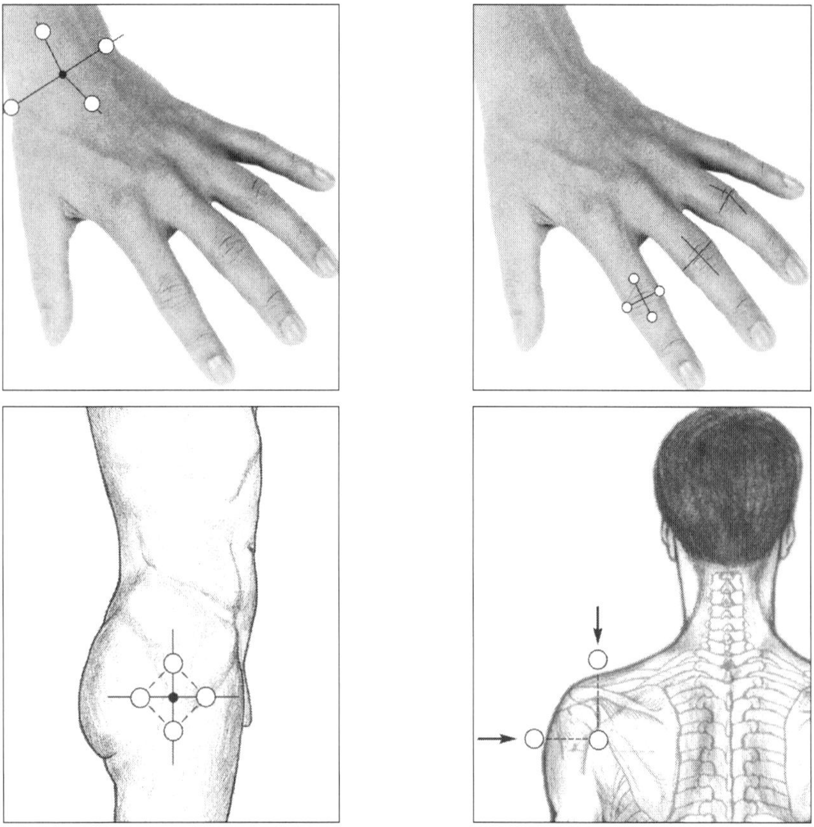

40 Joints: wrist, fingers, hip and shoulder

The symbolic meaning of a complaint

What is hidden behind a complaint? In my practice I am always alert to find the hidden causes of a client's complaint. I watch the reactions of a client during the treatment, since these are signals that can give an indication. In esogetic holistic medicine these reactions are called 'symbols', because they give a symbolic indication where the cause can be found.

Cramps in one's calf

Cramps in the calf are a good example of such a signal that contains a symbolic meaning. On the back of the leg, in the middle of the calf muscle – both left and right – lies a zone on the skin that Peter Mandel calls 'the zone of existence'. It has the oval shape of an ellipse. The left leg represents the emotional side and the right leg the rational, intellectual aspect of life.

Many people suffer from pain or cramps in the calves, which especially occur at night. The pain disturbs their rhythm of sleep, which leads to a chain reaction: disturbed sleep leads to more pain and more complaints.

Usually the pain is assumed to be caused by a lack of magnesium or a failure of the central nervous system. This may be correct, but at a deeper level these cramps are regarded in esogetic holistic medicine as a signal that something is amiss with the person's 'existence in the current moment'. If the pain is more dominant at the right side, this signifies that something is wrong in their daily life. If the pain is stronger on the left side, it indicates a disturbance of their 'emotional existence'.

I once treated a woman who had cramps in the calves from time to time. It didn't bother her too much, until her elder brother, who was a strong support for her, became seriously ill. The pain in her legs became so severe that there were days when she couldn't walk at all. Through the treatment of these zones she came to the insight that her existence was literally reeling. She needed to learn to walk on her own legs, because her brother couldn't support her any longer. This was the symbolic meaning.

CRAMPS IN ONE'S CALF

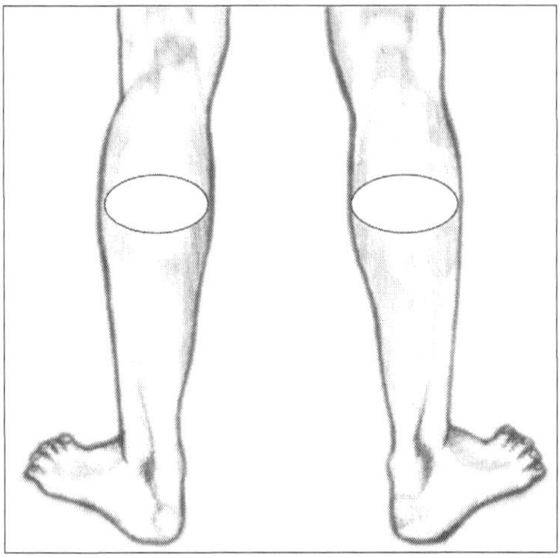

41 Cramp in one's calf: zone of existence

Location: in the middle of the calf. The zone has the shape of an ellipse with a height of about 2-3 FW and a width of 4-6 FW.

Sequence of treatment: Use the color orange and start on the left leg. Stroke the outline of the ellipse, starting from the top to the outside and coming back on the inside. Do the same on the right leg. Stroke the outline from the top to the outside. Treat both legs about 1 minute, this is on average 5 times the whole ellipse.

I advise people suffering from these cramps in the calves to treat these zones at home in the evening before going to sleep with the esogetic herbal oil. It has to be rubbed in vigorously and will enhance dream activity and regulate the sleeping rhythm. In dreams the unconscious, that contains absolute knowledge, opens up and offers help that is no longer heard or felt in daytime awareness. Something arises which Peter Mandel has called the 'resonance with the whole'. The complaints usually disappear quickly because the rhythm of life dynamics has been restored.

Once you start paying attention to the signals of the body and start understanding them, day by day your insight into your own being will increase. Slowly you start connecting with that which you have always known.

Everyone can treat these zones themselves in the evening, whether the calves are painful or not. It is also possible to combine this zone of existence with the treatment of the life stream points that is explained in the next section.

The life streams

Use the following treatment if you have any of the following symptoms:

- Feeling exhausted in the early morning
- Feeling weak and unwell
- When you notice that you age prematurely
- When recovering from a sickness

If you, or anyone in your family, notices such 'signals', it would be good to do this treatment on a daily basis for a while. Before I describe the treatment, I first give some information about the life streams according to Peter Mandel.

The concept of the life streams stems from the age-old Gilgamesh epic, which describes how God created man. God placed man in the Garden of Eden, where a river rose that branched out into four streams, all containing the 'Water of Life'. The meaning of this myth lies in the number 4, which in numerology is assigned to the Elixir of Life.

Peter Mandel used this ancient, esoteric knowledge to develop new therapeutic methods. In ancient times life was categorized in four temperaments and four elements, that arise from the number 5 and return to it. The four temperaments and the four elements – fire, earth, air and water – are the aspects that continuously create and destroy matter. They arise from the fifth element ether and return to it. The four streams containing the Water of Life are also connected with the four elements. They come from one stream, just as the four elements are subordinate to the ether. All that exists is connected to the number 4.

Already in the 2nd century B.C. the Roman scholar Claudius Galenus developed the theory of the temperaments. He distinguished four states of the human being: melancholic, choleric, sanguine and phlegmatic. These are the four temperaments. During his study of the colors Peter Mandel discovered the correlation between the colors and the four temperaments. The colors are red, yellow, green and blue. By assigning these four colors to the temperaments, new and fascinating possibilities for treatment opened up.

Peter Mandel has located the four life stream points on the body and tested them extensively in his clinic. In my own practice I also found that the treatment of these four points have a strong regenerating effect on people with degenerative diseases – it also helps to break through energetic blockages.

The meaning of the four life stream points

The color of the first life stream point is red, which corresponds with the choleric temperament. Indications for the first life stream point relate to vitality, regeneration of all psychosomatic complaints. The themes are: a free spirit, courage, attack, struggle, aggression, a drive to be independent, inventive creativity, the pursuit of the highest.

The second life stream point has the color of the phlegmatic temperament: green. The effect of this point and the color green is dissolving, detoxifying and eliminating. The characteristics of this temperament are: peaceful, gentle, humble, compassionate, strong in spirit, though sometimes lacking in self-confidence.

The third life stream point is the seat of the sanguine temperament and has the color yellow. The effect of this point is related to the lymphatic system – it strengthens and stimulates the flow of the lymph. The treatment of this point helps to strengthen the immune system. The control center of movement and power is also located in the area of the third life stream point. Therefore this point is also related to the muscular system and the joints. The sanguine temperament is social and charismatic, represents order and discipline, sacrifice, care and also the ego.

The fourth life stream point has the color blue and is connected to the melancholic temperament. All respiratory functions are related to it, also the lymph and the immune system. Number 4 symbolizes on the one hand: feeling excluded, the failure of one's desires and plans. On the other hand 4 also represents the struggle to take a spiritual step.

If you connect these four points diagonally, through the body, a new, fifth point is created. Peter Mandel regards this point as the center point of the human being: the center or source that we can long for with such intensity. This fifth point correlates with the other four and is influenced by the harmony or disharmony in one of the other points. If there is an irregularity in one of the four points, the fifth point is also out of balance.

These points return again and again in Peter Mandel's treatments. He calls them 'the four life streams of the human organism'. They play a special role in colorpuncture. The body always responds positively to the treatment of these points, whether treated with colorpuncture or massage.

Treatment of the life stream points combined with the zone of existence

Start this treatment with the zone of existence, followed by the four life stream points.

ZONE OF EXISTENCE

The center point of the 'zone of existence' lies in the middle of the calf. If we feel any pain or discomfort in our body, it is a sign that something is wrong in our life, in our existence. Treating this zone of existence can also provide an insight in the reason why there is pain. This insight may come in a dream, as a sudden flash or an intuitive 'knowing'.

Location of the zone: in the middle of the calf. The zone has the shape of an ellipse with a height of 2-3 FW and a width of 4-6 FW.

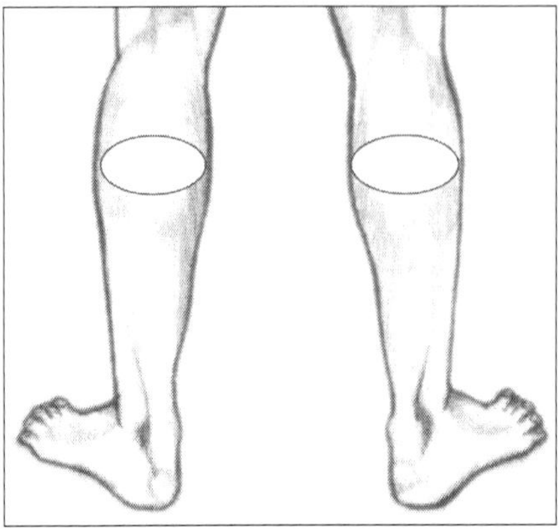

42 *Zone of existence*

Sequence of treatment: Use the color orange, starting with the left leg. Stroke the entire contour of the ellipse, starting at the top and moving to the outside. Do the same on the right leg, again stroking to the outside. Treat both legs for about 1 minute, on average that is 5 times the total ellipse.

LIFE STREAM POINTS

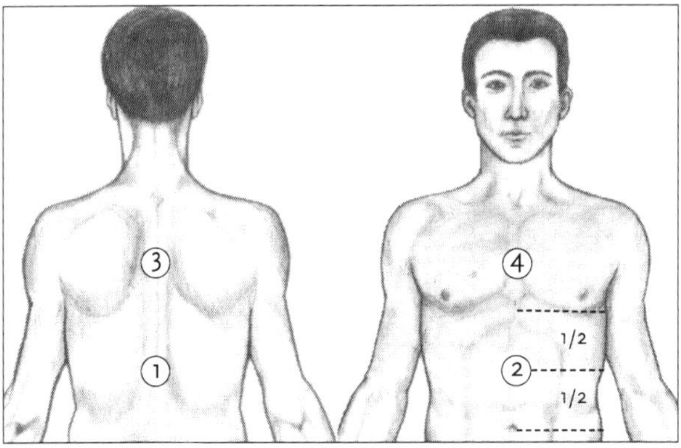

43 *The four life stream points*

1 = Life stream point 1 .... red
2 = Life stream point 2 .... green
3 = Life stream point 3 .... yellow
4 = Life stream point 4 .... blue

The location of the life stream points

Start by finding point 2. Once you have located it, it is easy to find point 1.

Point 2 = CV 12, which lies halfway between the navel and the lower tip of the sternum. Draw a imaginary horizontal line to the back of the body. Here, on the spine, point 1 is located.

Point 3 lies 1 FW up from an imaginary line connecting the armpits – in the middle on the spine. This is the third life stream point.

Point 4 lies in the middle of the sternum.

First massage point 1, 2, 3 and 4. Treat the points with the designated colors. Treat the points each for 30 seconds.

Finally massage a drop of the esogetic herbal oil on all four life stream points.

This treatment is best done just before going to sleep. After a while you will notice that your sense of well-being has improved.

Listening to the CD Immune Activity also gives a positive boost to your immune system. You can combine this sound therapy with all treatments that are described in this chapter.

If you feel there are underlying themes that you cannot yet recognize, esogetic sound therapy offers two other alternatives: the CD series Conflict Resolution or the series Totality: Body – Soul – Spirit.

8 Treatments especially suited for children

All children primarily need love, warmth, trust and security. A child should feel free to be authentic and should not be forced to live up to the expectations of the parents or caretakers. It reacts not so much to the words that are spoken, as to the tone of the voice, the intention, the love or attention that lies underneath the words.

Nowadays children are exposed at an early age to an avalanche of impressions from the outside world. Toddlers are taken to daycare or nurseries, watch TV and play video games. Many kids live in a state of tension, because their parents are fighting, are getting divorced or don't manage to spend enough time with them. These are just a few of the causes of stress in children.

On the other hand it is of great importance that a child is exposed to many different impressions in order to be able to develop his/her own individuality and talents. The parents' task is to find the golden mean – to allow the child to develop in a creative, but protected environment, while being aware of signals that indicate that the child gets overburdened.

Many treatments are available in colorpuncture that are suited for typical complaints that children have. I have selected three topics:

- Physical complaints, e.g.
  Inflammation of the ears and earaches
  Tonsillitis
  Returning colic or gripes in infants
  Sleeping disorders, restlessness
- ADHD, hyperactivity and lack of concentration
- Prenatal disturbances caused during pregnancy, birth traumas

Many children suffer from a lack of concentration, restlessness, hyperactivity, ADHD. The causes are innumerable and unique for each child. According to Peter Mandel they stem from a disturbance in the communication between the two brain hemispheres. In this chapter a few treatments are suggested that can be very effective.

For some children the trouble has started even before birth. It is not my intention to make mothers feel guilty. As a mother it is not an easy task to stay balanced during pregnancy or when mayor changes happen in life, e.g. your father dies, you lose your job, your partner leaves you or you have a car accident – of course you get emotional and temporarily lose your balance. A pregnant woman cannot always avoid stress, but it does influence the unborn child.

If the treatments listed under 'physical complaints' or 'hyperactivity and lack of concentration' do not have the desired effect on your child, you could try the prenatal treatment at the end of this chapter.

All treatments described in this chapter may be combined, although it is certainly not recommended to give them all at once. Peter Mandel often says: 'Less is more!' – short, simple treatments are often more successful than long, complicated ones.

Physical complaints

The lymphatic system as a psychological buffer

In the earlier chapters I have already pointed out the importance of the lymphatic system. Peter Mandel rates the lymphatic system as the highest priority, because it functions as a psychological buffer that absorbs any excess of emotional pressure. Whenever there is a reaction of the lymph, we can readily assume that the child has had an experience that caused stress. The body reacts via the lymphatic system in order to release the built-up tension.

Whenever the emotional tension becomes unbearable, it forms an emotional blockage, that holds the child in its grip. It cannot escape from it, the body cannot process all the impressions anymore and reacts with an infection. Therefore lymph treatments are always essential when we want to restore the physical balance. For a large part it is the lymph that takes care of the elimination of waste material from the body.

The first buffer area is the lymphatic system of the head: ears and tonsils.

Inflammation of the ear and earache

Indications: inflammation of the middle ear, earache.
Psychological indications: clinging and holding on, grinding one's teeth, not being able to let go.

Location of the points and sequence of treatment:

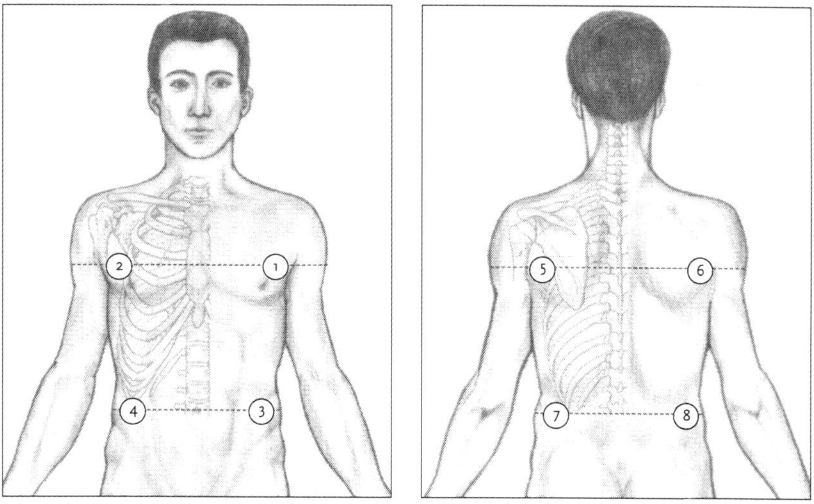

44 1st step: Inflammation of the ear and earache

1st step The drainage points of the lymph of throat and inner ear

1-8: Radiate each point 15 seconds in the sequence 1-8 ....violet

Location in front: points 1 and 2 are situated on the line that connects the armpits and 1 FW to the inside, on the side of the body. Points 3 and 4 lie on the same horizontal level as the navel, straight below points 1 and 2. The points on the back lie opposite the points on the front.

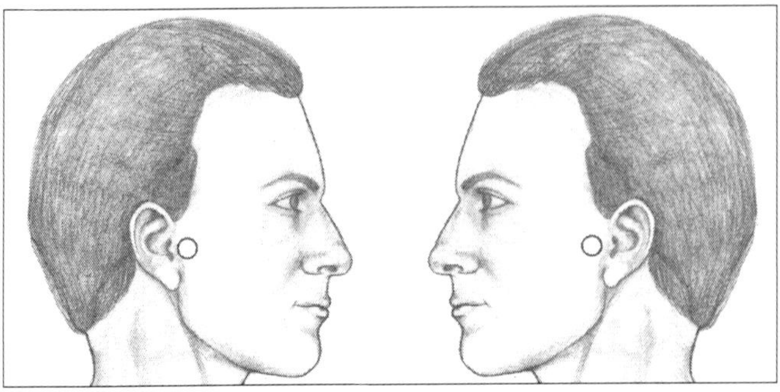

45 2nd step: Inflammation of the ear and earache

2ND STEP: TREATMENT OF THE GENERAL DRAINAGE POINTS OF THE LYMPH

Treat the points complementary ....violet/yellow

Location of the points: 1 FW in front of the auditory canal, on the maxillary joint of the jaw.

Complementary treatment: test the points for sensitivity. The more sensitive point is treated with violet, the less sensitive point with yellow. Treat both points for 15 seconds.

Acute or chronic tonsillitis

Children often have swollen glands. The parents are mostly advised to have a tonsillectomy done. That may be the right treatment in some cases, but not in all. Of course we have to consider that a chronic infection may have severe consequences. Often antibiotics are prescribed and taken over a long period of time. Children only benefit from antibiotics for a short period of time, because the antibiotics damage the intestinal flora, thereby weakening the immune system. A vicious circle starts and the complaints may well return quickly.

In each case the pros and cons have to weighed up, whether a tonsillectomy is the best remedy for a recurrent tonsillitis. In my opinion it is well worth trying to end this vicious circle. The following treatment often has miraculous results and can also be given as a preventive measure.

TONSILLITIS

Location of the points and sequence of treatment:

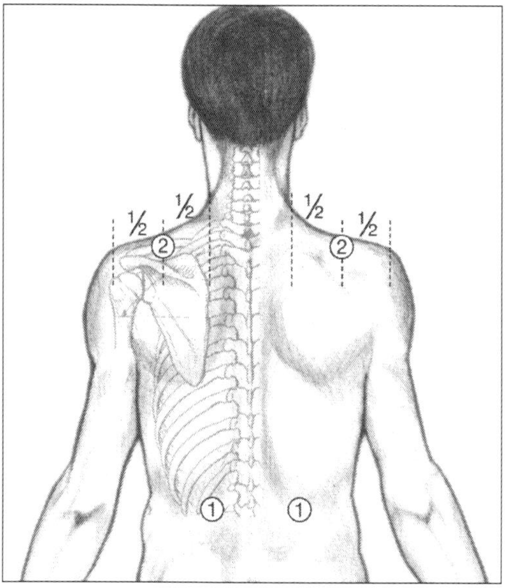

46 1st step: Tonsillitis

1ST STEP

1 = Kidney poles, first left, then right ....red
Location: we find the kidney poles in the angle of the 12th rib and the spinal protuberance of the first lumbar vertebra. Put your hands on your hips, place your thumbs against the lower ribs. Your thumbs will be on these points, which are always sensitive to pressure.

2 = Zones of the tonsils, first left, then right
In case of an acute tonsillitis ....yellow
In case of a chronic tonsillitis...red
Location: in the middle of the shoulders, slightly towards the back, lie the zones of the tonsils.

All points are treated for 30 seconds.

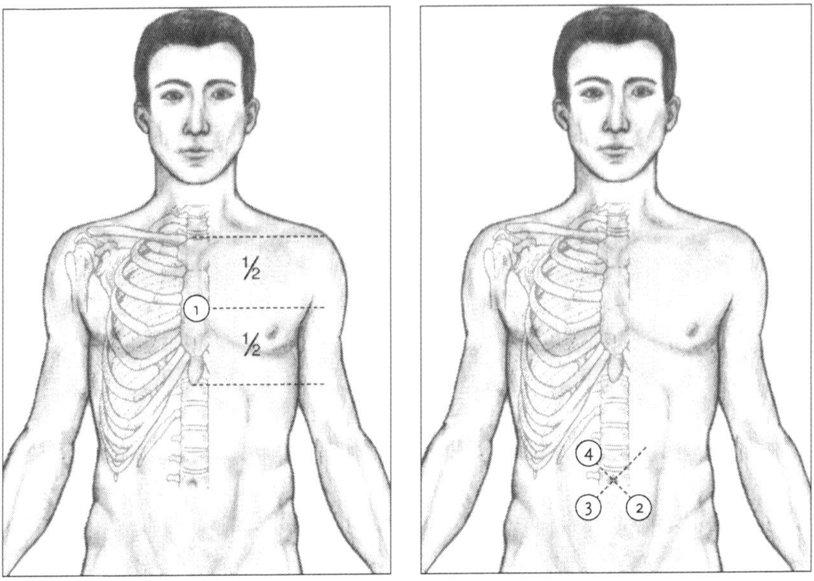

47 2nd step: Tonsillitis

2ND STEP

1 = Between CV 17 and CV 18, in the middle of the sternum .... violet
2-4 = Aggressive zones .... green
Locations of the zones: on a diagonal line 2 FW up from the navel, down, left and right.

We treat three of these four zones: the lower point on the left, the lower point on the right and the upper point on the right – in this sequence.

These aggressive zones, situated around the navel, form the lymph triangle that activates the flow of lymph in the belly. By treating these zones we stimulate the activity of the small and large intestine.

Peter Mandel calls them the aggressive zones, because the waste materials stored here can turn aggressive against us. By radiating them with green light we help the immune system to protect us against attacks from inside or outside.

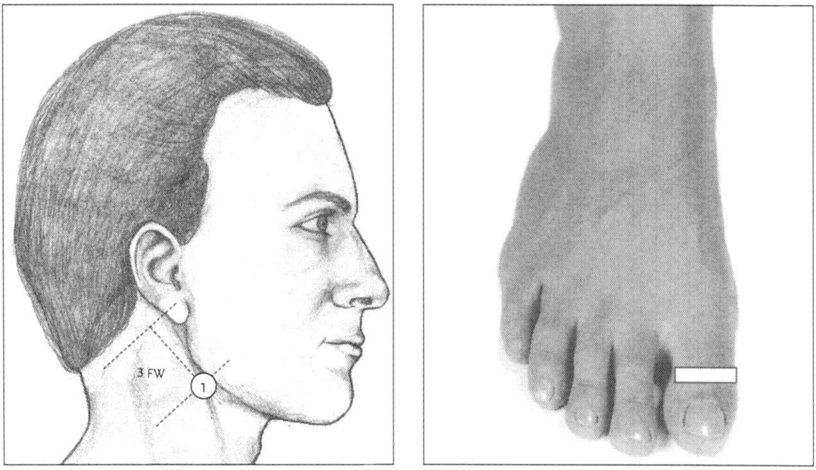

48 3rd step: Tonsillitis

3RD STEP

1 = Edge of the jaw
In case of acute complaints .... blue
In case of chronic complaints .... red
These points are located in the throat area, touching the jaw bone, left and right. Treat these points for 30 seconds.

2 = zone of the big toe, stroke from the inside to the outside and back, first left, then right .... red
These zones lie on the last joint of the big toe and relate to the cavities of nose and throat.

Disturbances in the lymphatic system can also be treated additionally by listening to the CD Immune Activity. This CD is also very helpful for adults.

Colic attacks or gripes in infants

This type of colic occurs especially in infants around the age of 3 months. For reasons unknown to science these infants suffer from abdominal pains. It could be an allergic reaction to a certain type of food that is new to the tiny body. The parents are worried and upset.

They suffer from lack of sleep, fear and anxiety dominate their lives. If there is no fever, vomiting or pallor, these colic attacks usually diminish after some time. Still, it is upsetting to see an infant cry so desperately.

> *A young mother with a crying baby came to my practice. The infant used to cry for hours after its meals. It was also crying when she came for the appointment. I immediately gave the treatment described below, which worked at once. The baby stopped crying, looked at the mother, started smiling and fell into a relaxed sleep. Then the mother started crying – such a relief!*

COLIC ATTACKS

1ST STEP COORDINATION 1

Location of the points and sequence of treatment:

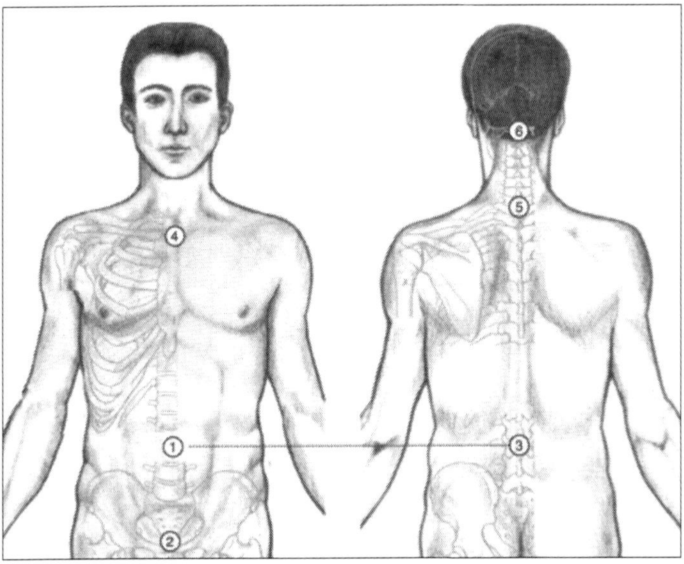

49 1st step: Colic attacks – coordination 1

1 = CV 8, the navel .... green
2 = CV 3, about 2 FW above the pubic bone, on the middle line .... orange

3 = On the back, on the spine, at the level of the navel..........violet
4 = CV 22, just under the throat, on the upper edge of the sternum in the hollow of the throat ....yellow
5 = GV 14, under the protuberance of the 7th cervical vertebra. When you feel along your neck, you find this cervical vertebra, that sticks out a bit..red
6 = GV 16, at the back of the head, in the hollow between the skull and the first cervical vertebra..................................blue

All points are treated 30 seconds.

2ND STEP AGGRESSIVE ZONES

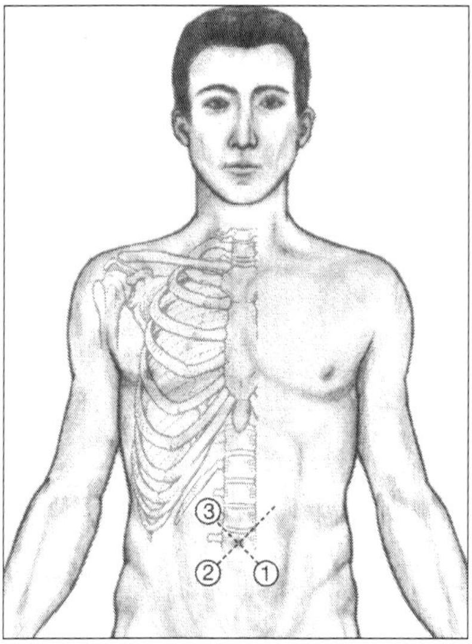

50 *2nd step: Colic attacks – aggressive zones*

1-3 = Aggressive zones ....green
Locations of the zones: on a diagonal line 2 FW up from the navel, down, left and right.
We treat three of these four zones: left down, right down and right up, in this sequence.

3RD STEP STOMACH DIAMOND

Indication: relaxation of the entire belly (can also be used for adults!).

Location and sequence of treatment:

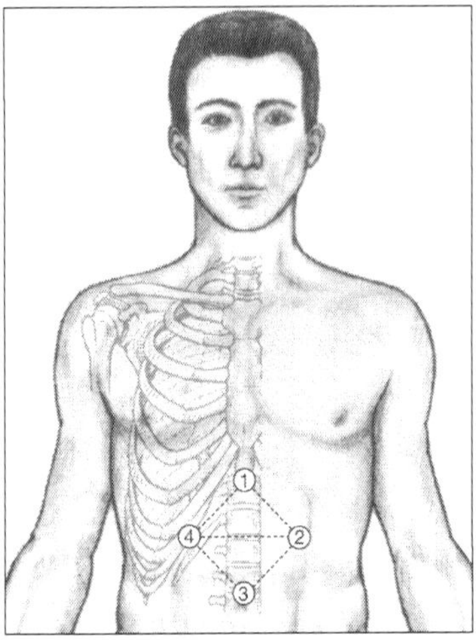

51 *3rd step: Colic attacks – stomach diamond*

1 = The tip of the sternum ....blue
2 = The 4 points form a rhombus. Point 2 and 4 are located on the horizontal line between point 1 and 3.....................blue
3 = On the upper edge of the navel..blue
4 = Opposite point 2...blue

Sleeping disorders

Children often suffer from sleeping disorders. Usually these are related to some fear: e.g. fear of darkness. In this context I would like to tell about a research done on the effect of light in the bedroom.

Richard Stone of the Scheie Eye Institute of the University of Pennsylvania in the US did research about the effect of light in the bedroom of small children. Many parents switch on a small light in the bedroom, because their children are afraid of the dark and cannot sleep. The eye nerve grows when it is light (in daytime), but if there is light in the night, the eye nerve continues to grow. This can lead to short-sightedness at a young age. Stone's research showed that:

- without a light in the bedroom 10% of the children were short-sighted.
- with a small bedroom light 34% of the children were short-sighted.
- in a fully-lit bedroom 55% of the children were short-sighted.

This type of short-sightedness disappears again when the children grow up.

His research is not completed yet. The researchers want to check if there are other causes as well. Their interim conclusion is that parents are advised not to leave any light on in the bedroom. Street lights in front of the window or other sources of light can also be disturbing. It is best if the bedroom is totally dark. As a compromise the parents could switch on a small light until the children are asleep and then switch it off. It would be best, though, not to leave any light on. The following treatment works well for sleeping disorders.

Sleeping disorders

Location and sequence of treatment:

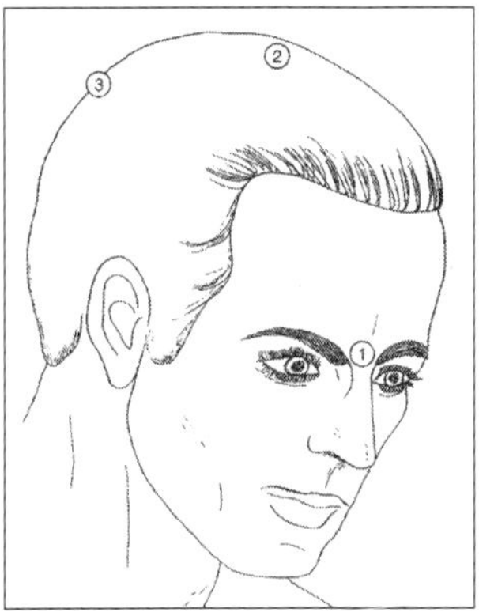

52 *Sleeping disorders*

1 = Yin trang, the point for the pineal gland, which lies between the eyebrows on the middle line .... blue
2 = GV 20: at the top of the head .... blue
Draw an imaginary line across the head between the tips of the ears, the point lies on the middle line of the body .... blue
3 = GV 19: 4 FW behind GV 20, at the point where the skull bends .... blue

The point yin trang activates the pineal gland, which influences the day-night rhythm. GV 20 and GV 19 relax the head.
All points are treated 30 seconds.

Restlessness

The restlessness that is connected with hyperactivity and ADHD will be discussed further on in this chapter. First I want to talk about the restlessness that is a temporary phenomenon, e.g. caused by something exciting the child will do that creates a certain nervousness or tension. It may be a school outing, a birthday party, an overnight stay with the grandparents. Or maybe it has been a hectic day with many impressions that the child has not been able to absorb and process. Here we treat the limbic system – a part of the brain that plays a major role in processing emotions.

RESTLESSNESS

1ST STEP

Location and sequence of treatment:

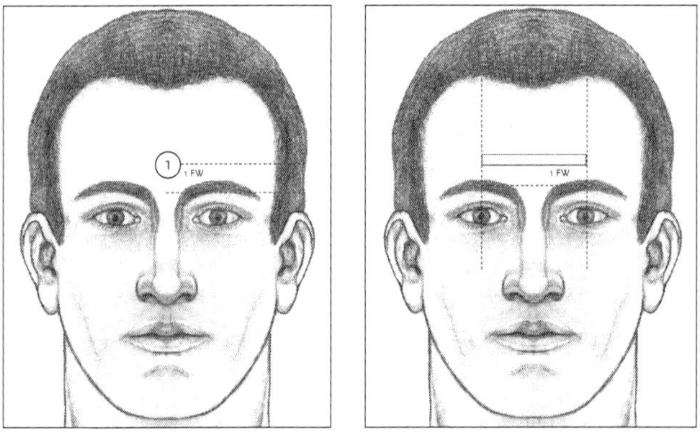

53 1st step: Restlessness

1 = The point for the limbic system, in the middle of the forehead, 1 FW above the eyebrows, 30 seconds.............yellow

2 = The neurasthenia line on the forehead, 1 FW above the eyebrows. The end of the line is located above the pupils of the eye (when looking ahead) ....violet
Stroke this line slowly back and forth, about 5 times.
The neurasthenia line has been explained in chapter 6. The point for the limbic system lies at the center point of this line.

2ND STEP

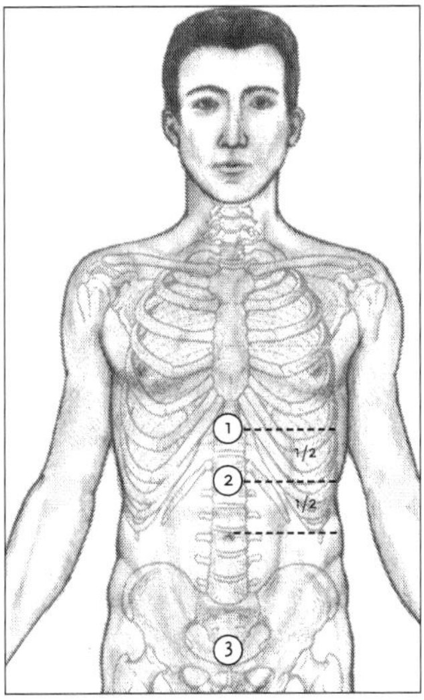

54 2nd step: Restlessness

Treat the following 3 points for 30 seconds.

1 = CV 14: 1 FW under the tip of the sternum ....blue
2 = CV 12: between the navel and the tip of the sternum ....blue
3 = CV 3: about 2 FW up from the edge of the pubic bone, on the middle line ....blue

A child with sleeping disorders can also benefit from listening to the CD Sleeping Disorders or the CD Psychosomatic Balance.

ADHD, hyperactivity and lack of concentration

In children – or adults – with hyperactivity, ADHD or lack of concentration the left and right hemisphere of the brain do not cooperate well. The right hemisphere rules the capacity to feel and the left one the rational thinking. Two other parts of the brain are also playing a part in this concerted action: the corpus callosum and the limbic system. The corpus callosum is the bridge between the left and the right hemisphere of the brain. The limbic system plays an important role in learning to deal with emotions and processing them. The functioning of the corpus callosum can get disturbed by traumas. These can be prenatal traumas or birth traumas, or e.g. a concussion as a result of a fall from a tree. Emotional events can also influence the functioning of the corpus callosum.

In the next treatment we aim to restore the balance between the two brain hemispheres and to heal the sustained traumas. It consists of a combination of well-known acupuncture points and others, which Peter Mandel discovered over the past decades of intensive treatment of his clients.

1ST STEP

INFORMATION BLOCKAGE TH 8

Th 8 (8th thoracic vertebra) has a special position on the body. It lies halfway the spine and forms the boundary between the upper and the lower part. The upper part also symbolizes the rational mind (the left brain hemisphere) and the lower part represents the capacity to feel (right brain hemisphere).

This treatment helps to connect the upper part with the lower part, the left side with the right side. Feeling is reconnected with thinking.

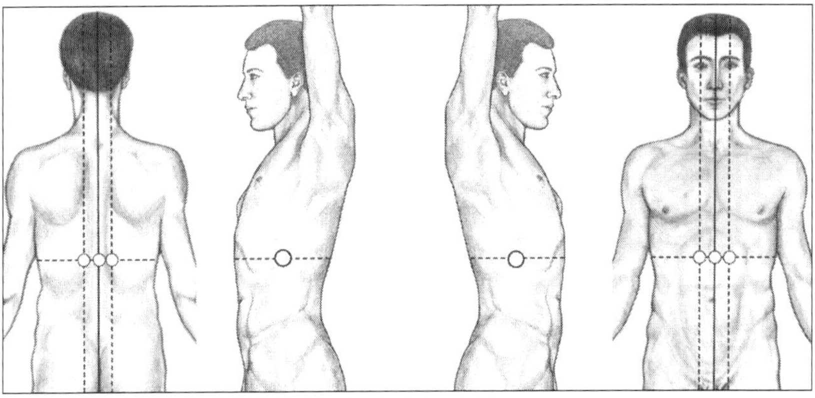

55 1st step: ADHD – information blockage Th 8

1 = Th 8 (8th thoracic vertebra): the center point of the spine on the back .... violet
2 = 1 FW from the center point to the left .... violet
3 = 1 FW from the center point to the right .... violet
4 = The point on the left side of the body .... violet
5 = The point on the right side of the body .... violet
6 = The tip of the sternum .... violet
7 = 1 FW from point 6 to the left .... violet
8 = 1 FW from point 6 to the right .... violet

All points are treated with violet. It is also possible to treat the points with turquoise. In that case give the complete treatment first with violet and the next time with turquoise.

All points are treated for 30 seconds.

2ND STEP

COORDINATION 1

Location of the points and sequence of treatment:

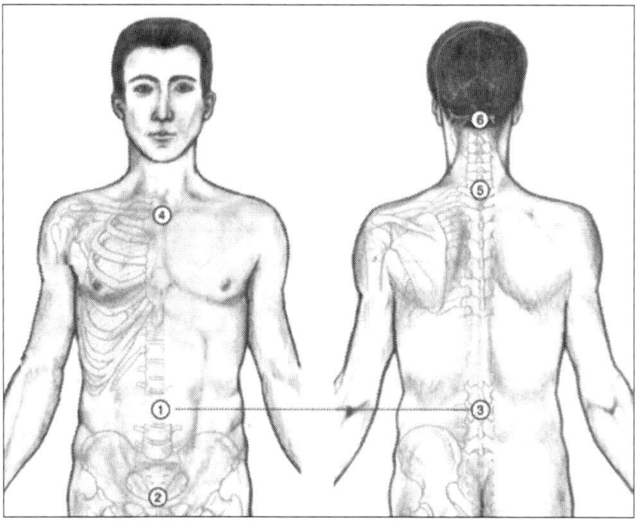

56 2st step: ADHD – coordination 1

1 = CV 8, the navel .... green
2 = CV 3, about 2 FW above the pubic bone, on the middle line .... orange
3 = On the back, on the spine, at the level of the navel .... violet
4 = CV 22, just under the throat, on the upper edge of the sternum in the hollow of the throat .... yellow
5 = GV 14, under the protuberance of the 7th cervical vertebra. When you feel along your neck, you find this cervical vertebra, that sticks out a bit........ red
6 = GV 16, at the back of the head, in the hollow between the skull and the first cervical vertebra........ blue

All points are treated 30 seconds.

These two treatments (information blockage Th 8 and Coordination 1) can be done consecutively in this sequence, in the beginning even daily.

After a while they can be alternated: day 1: Th 8, day 2: Coordination 1. You will probably find that the need for the treatments subsides. Whenever a situation occurs that the child becomes overactive, you can repeat the treatment.

ADDITIONAL THERAPY FOR ADHD, LACK OF CONCENTRATION OR LEARNING DIFFICULTIES

This is an additional treatment for ADHD, also to be used if the child suffers from lack of concentration or learning difficulties.

1ST STEP

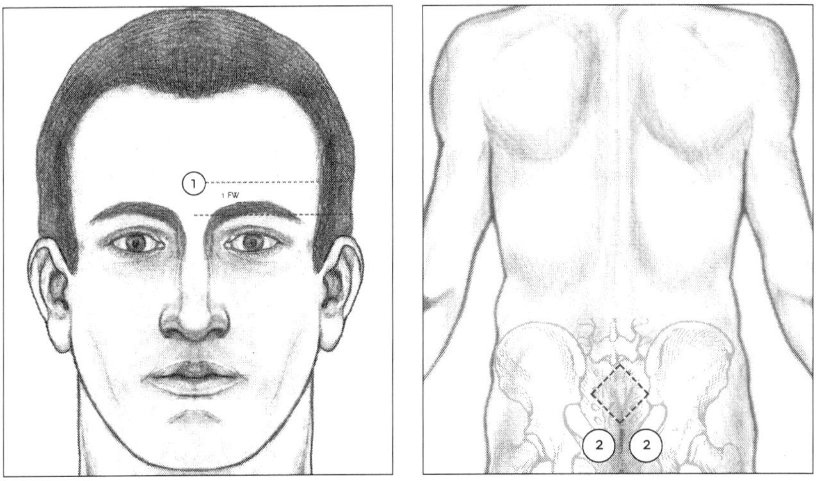

57 1st step: ADHD – additional treatment

1 = 1 FW up from yin trang ....yellow
This point influences the limbic system of the brain.

2 = 2 FW left and right of the center line of the body and 2 FW under GV 2. GV 2 is located at the beginning of the anal cleft. Treat complementary......................yellow/violet

Complementary treatment: test the points for sensitivity. The more sensitive point is given violet, the less sensitive point is treated with yellow.

With this treatment we reach the limbic system via the principle of the inverted man. This principle is explained in chapter 2.

2ND STEP

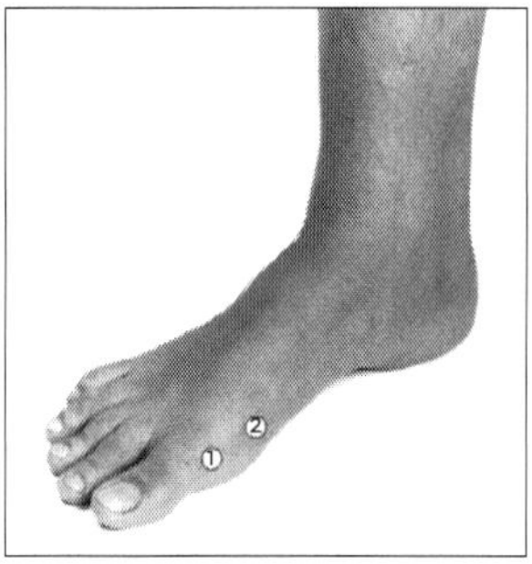

58 2nd step: ADHD – additional treatment

1 = SP 2: just in front of the main joint of the big toe ....yellow
This point lies on the stomach-pancreas meridian.
It promotes clarity in the head.

2 = SP 3: behind the main joint of the big toe........................yellow
Treat the points each for 30 seconds. First the left foot, then the right foot.

3RD STEP

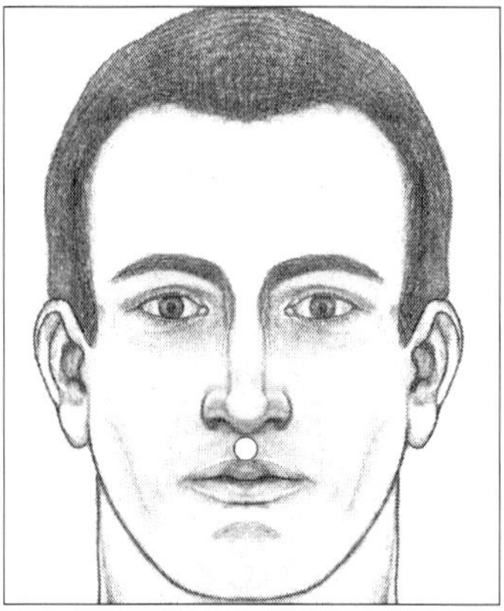

59 3rd step: ADHD – additional treatment

GV 26: a little up from the center point between upper lip and the bottom of the nose...yellow

GV 26 is the point for the corpus callosum. It helps to connect the right hemisphere (the emotional center) of the cerebrum with the left hemisphere (the rational center), and to improve the communication between the cerebrum and the brainstem. Emotion and rational mind, feeling and thinking, can thus be brought in balance. Right and left, upper part and lower part are harmonized.

Here is another tip for parents with hyperactive children: Ensure that the child's room has quiet colors, e.g. green or blue. Avoid the color red in the child's clothing or toys, as red will make it more active.

COORDINATION LINES ON THE FRONT AND BACK OF THE BODY

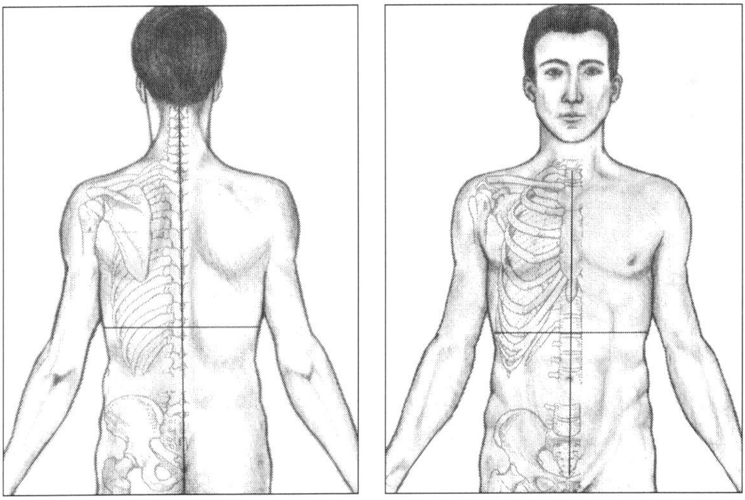

60 ADHD – coordination lines

First stroke the coordination lines on the back:
Vertically..violet
Horizontally..yellow

Then stroke the coordination lines on the front:
Vertically..yellow
Horizontally..violet

Location: First locate the center point on the front side: this is life stream point 2 (CV 12), between the navel and the tip of the sternum. The center point on the back is life stream point 1, opposite CV 12 on the spine.

Procedure: stroke the vertical lines slowly with full attention 3 times up and down. Start at the top and stroke down, then up again. This counts as 1 time, repeat this 2 times. Then stroke the horizontal lines: start on the left side and stroke to the right and back again. This counts as 1 time, repeat this 2 times.

This is a wonderful aid for anyone who is out of balance and can be used as an addition to the other ADHD treatments. This too restores the communication between left and right, front and back.

Children who have difficulties learning or have problems with concentration benefit from wearing yellow glasses. They can wear them while doing their homework.

Many children profited as well from listening to the CDs Motivation or Concentration. Parents reported to me that even the teachers at school were impressed by the improved powers of concentration of children who regularly listened to these CDs.

Traumas

All children get traumatized occasionally. A fall in the school yard, being teased by other children, the death of a pet – many small or big events can leave a mark.

The following trauma treatment helps to restore the communication between the left and right brain hemisphere, to relax the mind and dissolve the tension the child has incurred. This treatment also works well for adults who have sustained traumas in their life. It helps to release the tension that has remained as a result of the trauma.

I once treated a woman who suffered from headaches. While I was treating these points with colored light, she started relating her experiences as a child in a Japanese concentration camp. She said: 'Now I can suddenly see that I have always felt so constrained, it must be related to that experience.' Seeing clearly the connection between her traumatic experiences in childhood and her headaches helped to decrease the headache. It had lightened her burden.

TRAUMAS

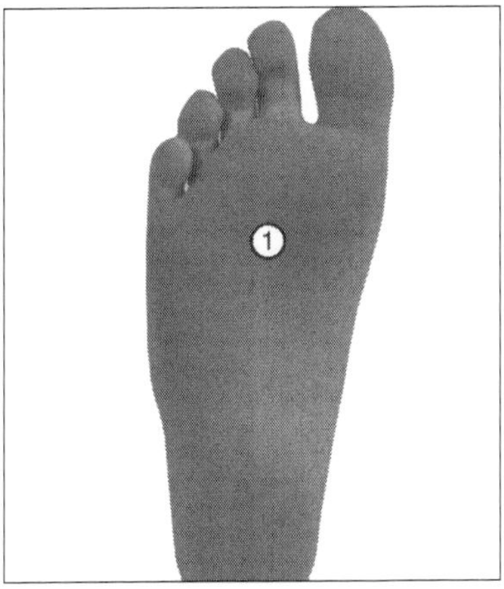

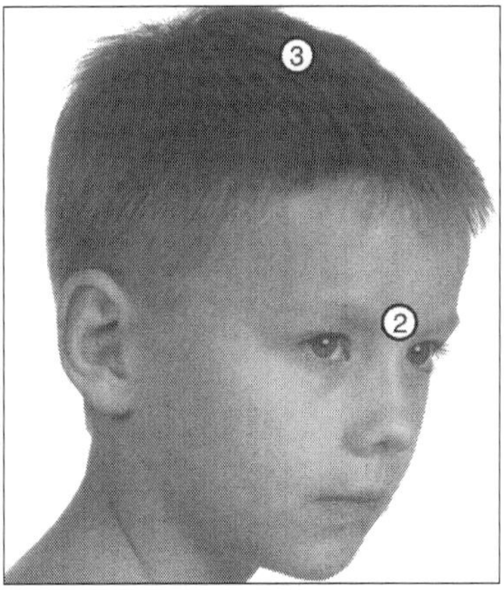

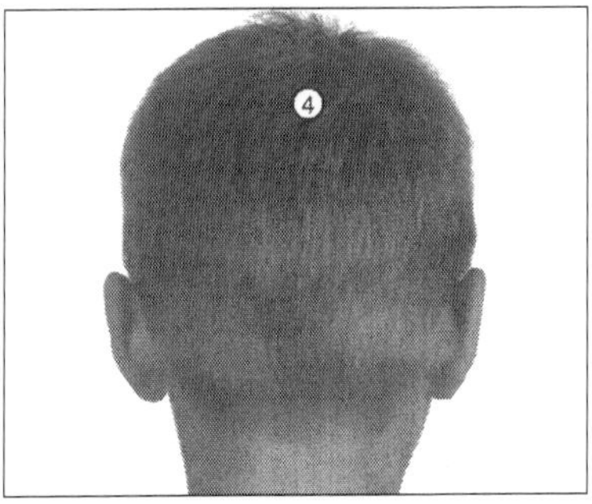

61 Traumas

1 = KD 1 .... red
KD 1: is located on the sole of the foot, between the 2nd and 3rd toe, in an indentation that is found when the toes are bent. Left and right.

2 = Yin trang, in the center between the eyebrows .... violet
Yin trang is the coordination point of the pineal gland.

3 = GV 20 .... violet
GV 20: on the top of the head. Draw an imaginary line over the head from one tip of the ear to the other. The point lies on the middle line of the body.

4 = GV 19 .... violet
GV 19 lies 4 FW behind GV 20 on the middle line, where the skull bends down.

The violet glasses also assist children who are processing traumas.

Prenatal colorpuncture

The prenatal therapy originates from Robert St. John's metamorphosis therapy.

St. John had discovered that there is a line on the inside of the foot that corresponds with the nine months of pregnancy. He developed a special massage technique for this line and also used it on lines on the hands and the head. His method proved extremely successful, especially with handicapped children. In England he was quite famous and held in high esteem for this healing method.

Many years ago Peter Mandel became familiar with St. John's method and he experimented with the use of colors on this line, because he was convinced that light and color transmit pure information. He assumed that the original information given to us before birth, is disturbed by emotional imprints and patterns we absorb during pregnancy and at birth. He called this line the line of the spirit and added two more lines: the line of the soul and the line of the body.

In this way the treatment was complete in Mandel's view, because now soul, spirit and body were all included in the therapy. The spirit line represents a time line from conception till birth. The first week of pregnancy is found at the big toe and birth is situated at the back of the heel. The same principle applies to the other lines.

This theory is based on the premise that the fetus in the womb absorbs all the experiences of the mother, both her inner emotions and the influence of her surroundings. Any negative experiences before birth can especially leave traces in later life.

Of course positive experiences also influence the unborn child. If the mother is happy and full of joy during pregnancy, it has an important effect. There are many examples of mothers who used to listen to classical music during pregnancy and bore a child with a musical gift. Modern medical and neurological research has shown that the limbic system is already fully developed after the first six weeks of pregnancy. This indicates that the fetus can already register and store emotions or feelings a month and a half after conception.

According to Peter Mandel traumas from those early days influence our life later on and can lead to sickness or weakness. In the beginning these weak links will not yet be so obvious, but later in life insolvable problems or repetitive conflicts may emerge.

The following treatment may be given from the age of 1, or even just after the baby is born, if it is clear that there have been complications during pregnancy or birth. Prenatal colorpuncture is also a good treatment for adults. We all carry impressions from our time in the womb that still determine our day-to-day life.

Whenever I give prenatal colorpuncture treatments, I notice that almost everyone who receives the treatment sinks into a state of deep relaxation. At a deep level unconscious and subconscious tensions seem to dissolve automatically. I once treated a 80-year old woman, who felt she still carried the impressions of the 1st World War in her system (that was literally what she said). She was born in 1917.

BASIC TREATMENT PRENATAL COLORPUNCTURE

The first step is to stroke the prenatal line according to St. John, which Peter Mandel has named the spirit line. Start at the joint of the big toe (spleen/pancreas meridian) and slowly stroke in an arch to the highest point towards the back of the heel and then back to the toe. This counts as 1, repeat this 2 more times.

The spleen/pancreas meridian runs as a dividing line over the inside of the foot. Sometimes this boundary is visible as the division between what in Chinese medicine is called the 'red and the white flesh'. It can also be distinguished by the lines and wrinkles on the foot. The stronger wrinkles are visible on the bottom of the foot, close to the sole, and the finer ones are on the upper part of the foot. This can be seen even in babies. The spleen-pancreas meridian runs up on the inside of the ankle, but we extend the line to the back of the heel.

The second step is stroking the soul line. Start stroking from the nail bed of the third toe up to acupuncture point ST 41 and back. This counts as 1, repeat this 2 more times. ST 41 lies in the indentation of the foot, in the hollow.

The third step is stroking the body line. We start at acupuncture point UB 67. UB 67 lies at the nail bed of the little toe, on the outside, and here too one can observe clearly the difference in color on the side of the foot. We follow the arch to the highest point and end at the back of the heel, where the first line also ended. Stroke back to the starting point and repeat 2 more times.

Location of the lines and sequence of treatment:

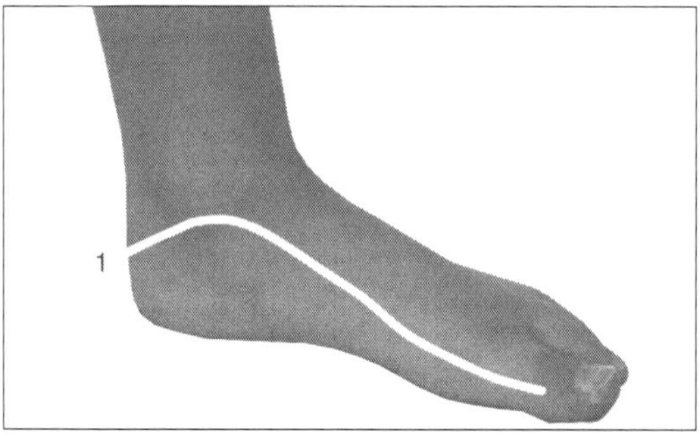

62 *Prenatal treatment: spirit line*

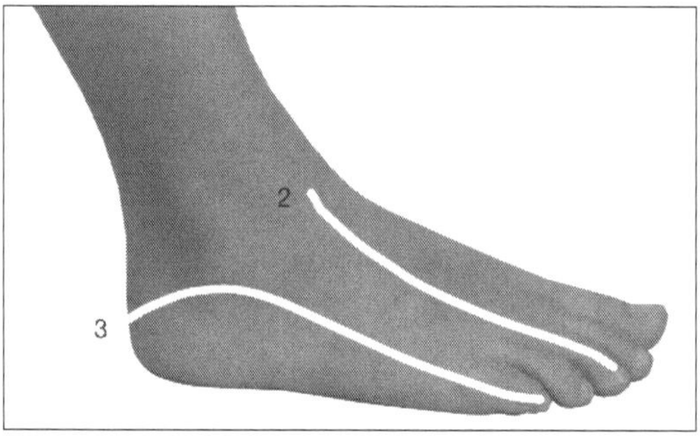

63 *Prenatal treatment: soul line and body line*

Stroke the spirit line on the inside of the foot............................violet
Stroke the soul line on top of the foot ....orange
Stroke the body line on the outside of the foot.........................yellow

The stroking should be done slowly and with a feeling of tranquility. First stroke the three lines on the left foot and afterwards the three lines on the right foot. Then the treatment is complete.

This treatment may be given once a week and in total up to ten times, if you feel it is needed. The child will indicate when it is sufficient, because the complaints will disappear. He/she will become more quiet or rather less shy, he/she may suddenly start playing with other children or have a better sleep. If the child is old enough to talk, pay attention to what he/she tells, let the child make a drawing, play with clay or paint. You can also ask the child to talk about his/her experience during the treatment, while it is given or the next day. This feedback may give an insight in the background of the problem.

If you give this treatment to adults or to yourself, it is helpful to watch which thoughts, images or memories come up, both in yourself and in the persons you treat. You may find some themes that are still running in their lives.

As I already mentioned, this treatment can also be applied to very tiny infants. If there have been problems during pregnancy or at birth, it is a valuable aid.

Most people that receive this treatment respond by going into a state of deep relaxation. I often hear comments like: 'At last I feel more at home in my body' or: 'Now I finally feel I really want to be here'.

Tanja is 41 years old. She came to me with complaints about her bronchial tubes and her skin. She often suffered from eczema. She told me that straight after birth her body was covered with eczema. It had disappeared after a while, but her skin remained a weak link. Because she had skin rashes straight after birth, I gave her a few prenatal treatments. She reacted well to them, had more energy, her skin looked clearer, but the main benefit for her was the feeling of having 'landed' on this earth without having to fight continuously. During the treatments she connected with a deep-rooted feeling of always being in a struggle. And she didn't even know what she was struggling with! It gave her a feeling of liberation and relief to be free from this struggle.

Deidre, a girl of around 2 years, suffered from coughs, colds and a runny nose. Her doctor was considering to have her tonsils removed. I combined tonsillitis treatments with the prenatal treatment, because her mother told me she found it difficult to be a single mother. As soon as she got pregnant, her partner had broken off the relationship and didn't want anything to do with her or the child. Deidre started playing with other children in the daycare center after the treatment, even though earlier she had had much trouble making contact. The tonsils did not need to be removed.

9

Treatments for stomach, liver, gallbladder and intestines

Stomach

When we mention the stomach our first thought is of food. 'We are what we eat', is an old Chinese saying. Wrong eating habits can lead to acidification of the body. This acidification and an overdose of stress are the main cause of stomach complaints. If we want to have a well functioning stomach and intestinal tract we should first of all keep a close watch on our eating habits. We need to eat sufficient fibers, chew well and slowly and ensure that our meals contain the right balance between acid and base contents.

Our meals in the West usually contain a large amount of acid forming nutrients such as meat, sugar, cheese and very few base forming ingredients. Base forming ingredients are raw vegetables and fruits. By eating more of these we can improve our internal environment. If we can create a proper inner balance – both physically and psychologically – we have less trouble 'digesting' the more difficult challenges in life and don't need to disturb our stomach by eating the wrong foods.

The stomach is also an organ that stores emotions. We could even say it is a 'feeling' organ. We often keep on eating or snacking, thus overloading the stomach, because we don't want to feel a negative emotion that comes up, e.g. fear, loneliness, boredom, sadness or anger. We tend to drown unpleasant feelings in our body by eating, drinking or smoking. Our bodies give us a signal in such moments, inviting us to have a good look at what we really need, to feel what is lacking in our lives. If we don't observe these needs and try to chase our unpleasant feelings away by eating, we overburden our bodies even more and end up further away from a solution.

The stomach is a fairly sturdy organ, but it is quite sensitive to stress. 'He couldn't stomach it' is an expression for not being able to digest a negative emotion. When these emotions and problems accumulate and don't get processed, one is likely to get a stomach ulcer or other stomach complaints.

The daily stress that we experience 24 hours – day and night – accumulates in the solar plexus. Peter Mandel had to conclude that many diseases result from such accumulated tensions, resulting in an incapacity of the stomach to digest food, which leads to acidity. If internal tensions are not resolved, we take the pressure with us in our sleep. This permanent level of tension leads to a permanent state of acidity. Over the years the mucous membrane of the stomach is affected and the acid/base balance is badly disturbed, leading to the first physical complaints.

Stress can also be caused by a mind-related existential struggle or the permanent desire to achieve more, to possess more, to experience more. We chase an unachievable goal and feel increasingly frustrated. This internal struggle is mainly a conflict between feeling and rational thinking. If the rational mind is mostly on top, the stomach gets disturbed.

When the internal pressure is building up, the following treatment of the indicated zones and points offers the possibility to let go of tension and stay healthy, thereby preventing serious complaints at a later stage.

Stomach – preventive measures

You can settle your stomach by:
- Touching and massaging
- Connecting with your feeling
- Meditating, reflecting, contemplating, rather than worrying and being anxious.

Earlier in this book the color blue is described as being the color of peace and infinity. This cool color has a calming effect. These relaxing and calming properties of the color blue are used to relieve headache and migraine, as well as stomach aches, muscle cramps and certain heart conditions. Blue instills tranquility and silence, it helps you to come back home to yourself. One way to bring relaxation is to stroke the entire gastric region with the color blue.

Yellow stimulates the metabolism, the glands and the production of gastric juices. After overeating or if your metabolism is slow, it is helpful to stroke the stomach with yellow.

Choose either blue or yellow for your treatment, do not combine them. Stroke the stomach for 1 minute.

Some more options:

ZONE OF THE SOLAR PLEXUS

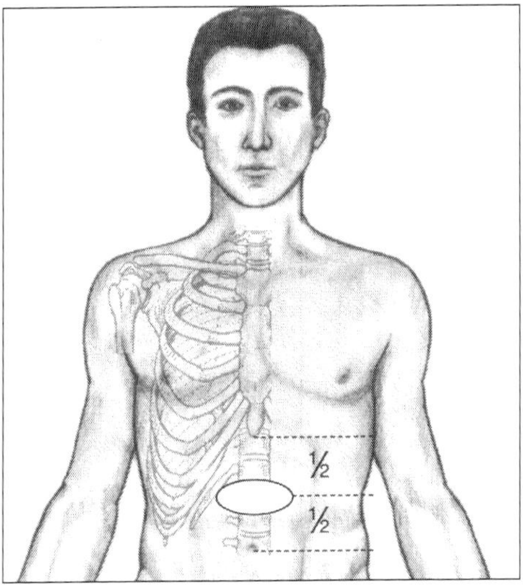

64 *Zone of the solar plexus*

Under the sternum lies the zone of the solar plexus. It is about the size of your hand. Before going to sleep, lie down on the bed, pull up your legs, close your eyes and softly massage this area, progressively going deeper into the stomach. Massage until you feel a slight pain, then stop. Rub three drops of the esogetic herbal oil on the area.

TWO ZONES IN THE LEFT SHOULDER AREA

Draw two imaginary crossing lines to divide the left shoulder blade into four parts. By pressing lightly on the inner upper section you will find a sensitive spot. This is zone 1 and it is always sensitive, even if there are no complaints. Peter Mandel calls it the zone of the problems that we carry. Massage this point until you reach the pain barrier. Rub a drop or two of the esogetic herbal oil on it. If you apply colorpuncture, the zone may be treated for 30 seconds with the color blue.

Zone 2 is directly related to the stomach. This zone lies between the left shoulder blade and the spine, at the height of the middle of the shoulder blade. Treat this zone the same way you treated zone 1: massage, rub in a few drops of the esogetic herbal oil and apply the color blue for 30 seconds.

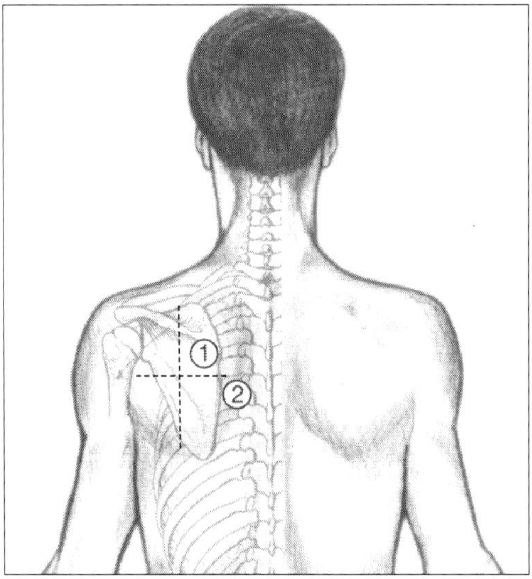

65 *Zones on and next to the left shoulder blade*

Tension in the stomach and the upper belly

The following treatments can be applied if you feel tension in the upper belly. They bring feeling and thinking into harmony, relax the solar plexus, dissolve blocked emotions and balance a disturbed rhythm of sleep. These two treatments can be given in sequence.

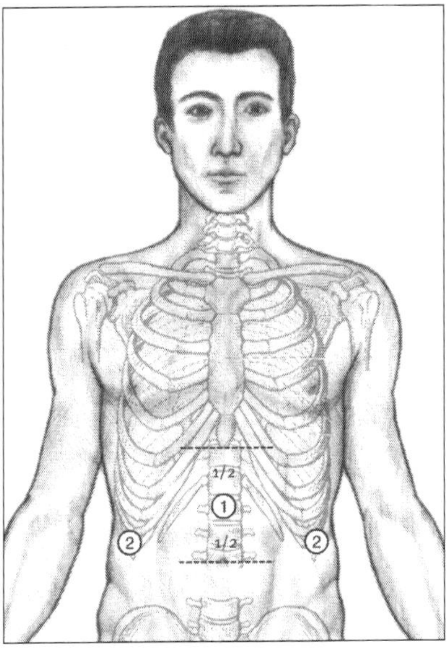

66 *Opening the solar plexus 1*

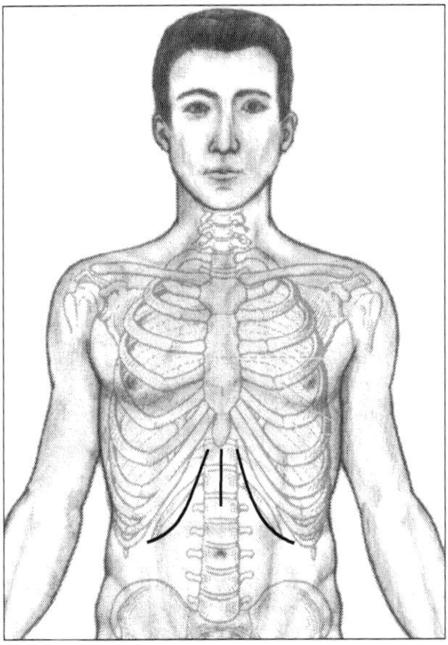

67 *Opening the solar plexus 2*

Opening the solar plexus 1

Location and sequence of treatment:

1 = CV 12: between the navel and the tip of the sternum ...... yellow
2 = LI 13: at the end of the ribcage, on the tip of the 11th rib, first left, then right .... yellow

Opening the solar plexus 2

Location and sequence of treatment:

1 = On the left side of the body, stroking along the ribcage from the tip of the sternum till 11th rib .... violet
2 = On the right side of the body, stroking along the ribcage from the tip of the sternum till 11th rib .... yellow
3 = From CV 12 (between the navel and the tip of the sternum) up to the tip of the sternum .... yellow

Stroke each line 5 times back and forth.

EMOTIONAL TENSION

The following treatment works well if you feel tension in the upper belly that is connected with stress and emotions.

Location and sequence of treatment:

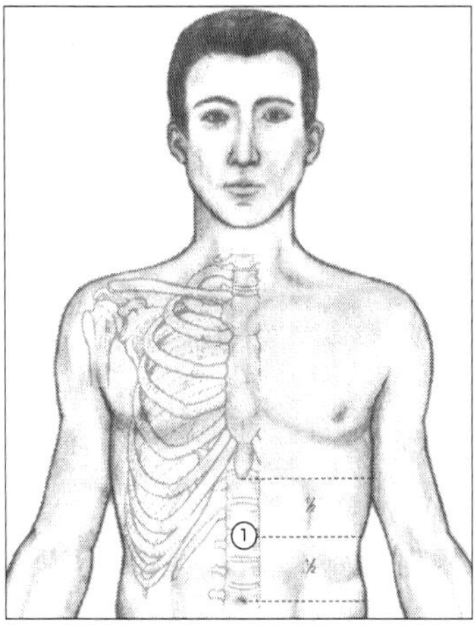

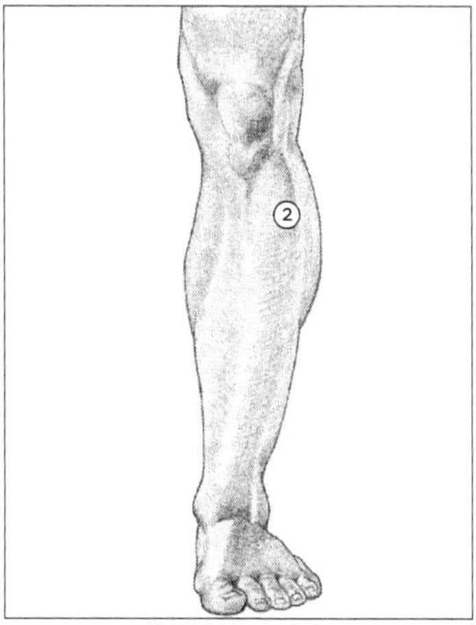

68 1st step: Emotional tension

1ST STEP

1 = CV 12, between the navel and the tip of the sternum ......yellow
2 = ST 36, on the outside of the calf, treat complementary ....blue/orange

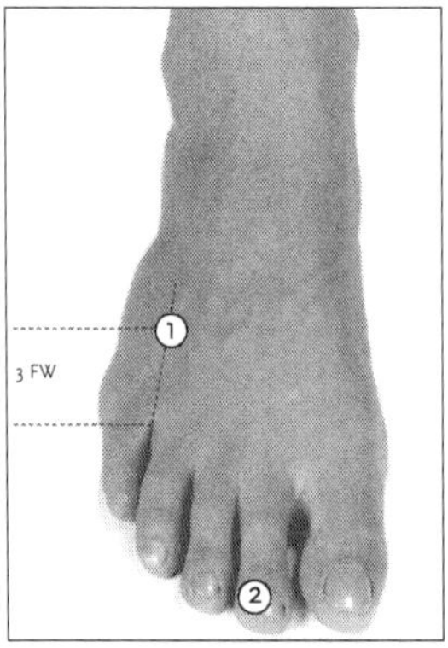

2ND STEP

1 = GB 41: halfway between the top of the outer ankle and the webbing between the 4th and 5th toe ....yellow
2 = ST 45: on the cuticle of the 2nd toe, towards the 3rd toe, treat complementary....................yellow/violet

69 2nd step: Emotional tension

Listening to the CD Psychosomatic Balance gives an extra support.

Diana has her own light set and sometimes comes to me for a check-up. I give her a treatment and homework, so she can continue to treat herself at home. When she visited me recently, she told that she has stomach complaints from time to time. She noticed an uneasy feeling in her stomach, sometimes after meals or in between meals during the day. It helped her to rub her belly with her hand, but she was a bit concerned about it. She also had heartburn at times. Her complaints began about three months earlier. She had started to worry about the economic recession and wondered if she too would lose her job. Her worries increased. During the treatment a memory surfaced of her father, who had once lost his job and after a few difficult months had found a new, better job that he was happy with. Suddenly she realized that redundancy might open up new opportunities for her. There was no need to worry.

The homework I gave her was to treat the gastric region with blue and to give herself the treatment for emotional tension described earlier. She could now treat herself if worries would surface again.

Liver and gallbladder

The liver lies on the right side of the upper belly, partly under the ribcage. The liver is essential for the metabolism and cleanses the blood by breaking down the toxic waste. The gallbladder stores the bile that is needed to digest fat.

In esogetic medicine much emphasis is given to the feelings that belong to the organs. In chapter 4 I already gave some examples. Psychologically liver and gallbladder are considered to be the organs that are related to strong emotions.

Liver and gallbladder are connected to the following emotions:

- Excitement, impatience
- Dramatizing, the inability to adjust
- Anger, irritation
- Being indecisive, having trouble taking decisions

Positive emotions related to these organs are:

- Being dynamic and active
- Stating clearly who you are and expressing yourself
- Being original and unique
- Tension and relaxation

The less pleasant, negative emotions are signals that can give a warning that liver complaints are pending. A cramp or pain in the liver area or tension that leads to pain in the right shoulder or at the right side of the neck are such physical warnings. The gallbladder lies on the right side of the belly and leads to complaints on that side. Complaints on the right side of the neck indicate gallbladder afflictions, as the gallbladder meridian runs along the back of the neck.

We can give ourselves preventive treatments to relieve the pressure on liver and gallbladder, which will also give us more space on the mental plane. It is good to take note of your emotions before and after such a treatment.

The best time for these treatments is at night before going to sleep.

Liver and gallbladder – preventive treatments

1. Massage the right upper region of the belly and apply a hot compress.

   Massage the right upper region of the belly. Prepare a hot compress by wrapping a damp towel around a hot water bottle and place it on that area. Lie down with the compress for 15 minutes. Afterwards rub 3 drops of esogetic herbal oil on the liver area.

2. Treating the area with color – two options

   - Yellow, if you want to stimulate the function of liver and gallbladder or if you experience strong emotions. Stroke the area with yellow for 1 minute.
   - Violet, if you want to relieve physical tension or pain. Stroke the area with violet for 1 minute.

LIVER AND GALLBLADDER SEGMENTS ON THE BACK

Between the spine and the edge of the right shoulder blade one often finds hard muscle cords. This is the area where signals of the liver manifest. On the right side of the neck lies the segment of the gallbladder. It is an area where tension accumulates and sometimes pain is felt, even if the gallbladder itself does not give complaints. Both zones can be massaged and rubbed with 3 drops of esogetic herbal oil. They can also be treated with light and color. Both zones are treated with yellow for 30 seconds.

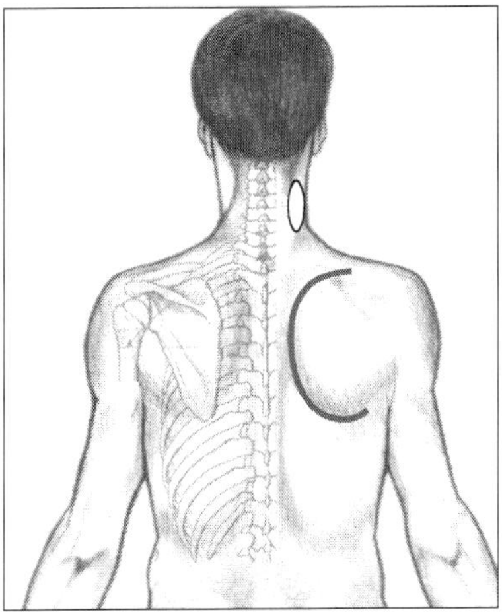

70 *Liver and gallbladder segments*

Gallbladder complaints after overeating

Many people have a weak gallbladder, sometimes resulting in a nagging pain in the upper right part of the belly, at times accompanied with a pain that radiates in the right arm. After eating the wrong food, overeating or an intake of too much fat, these complaints can flare up.

The following treatments can give a quick and effective relief, not only when the pain is acute, but they can also be used as a preventive measure. If you suffer regularly from these complaints, I suggest you apply these treatments once a week.

GALLBLADDER TREATMENT 1

Location and sequence of treatment:

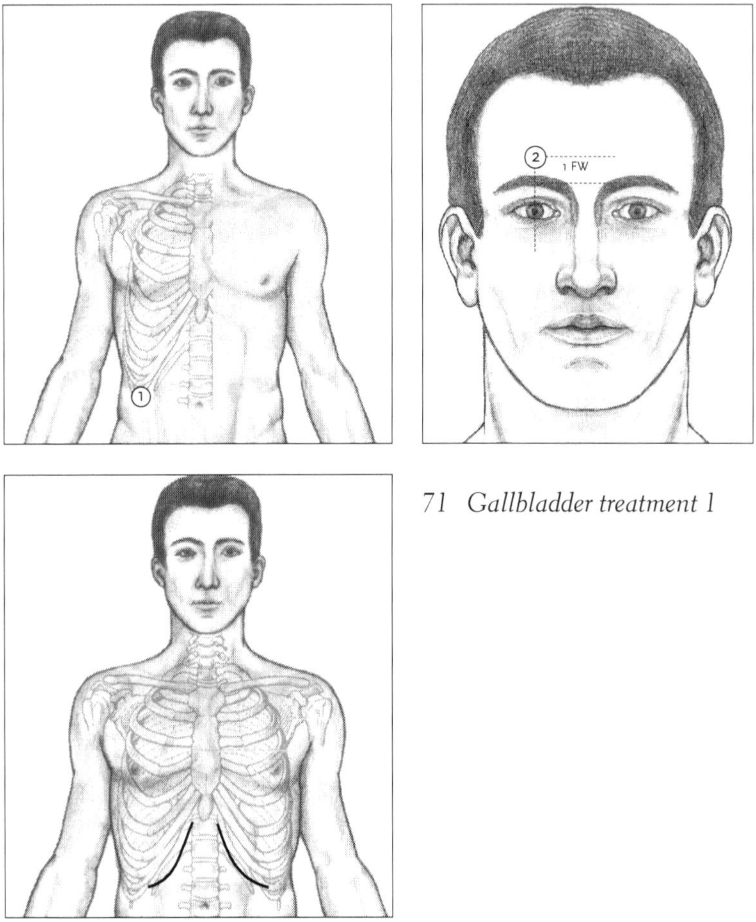

71 Gallbladder treatment 1

1 = LV 13 at the end of the ribcage – on the tip of the 11th rib, only on the right side .... yellow

2 = GB 14: 1 FW above the eyebrow on a vertical line up from the pupil (when looking straight ahead), only on the right side .... yellow

3 = Stroke the costal arches 3 times back and forth
Right side .... yellow
Left side .... violet

GALLBLADDER TREATMENT 2

Location and sequence of treatment:

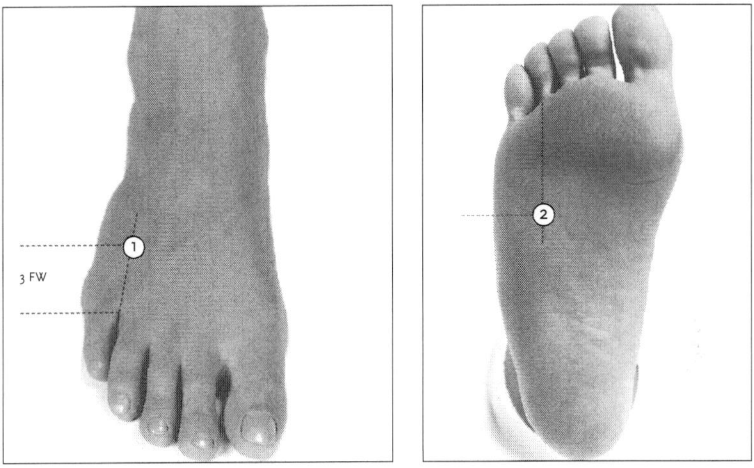

72 *Gallbladder treatment 2*

1 = GB 41: halfway between the top of the outer ankle and the webbing between the 4th and 5th toe ....yellow

2 = Zone of the gallbladder on the sole of the foot ....yellow
This point lies 'opposite' GB 41.

Points 1 and 2 are only treated on the right side.

Treatment 1 and 2 for the gallbladder can best be done in sequence.

The CDs that support this treatment are: the series Totality: Body – Soul – Spirit.

Treatment for gallbladder complaints

The following treatment can be applied in case of a gallbladder colic pain, or a gallbladder related migraine (i.e. a migraine on the right side of the head, usually starting at the right side of the neck).

If you have a weak gallbladder or have regular complaints, I suggest you massage the following points daily before going to sleep. After massaging them, rub 1 or 2 drops of esogetic herbal oil on the points.

GALLBLADDER COMPLAINTS

Location of the points and sequence of treatment:

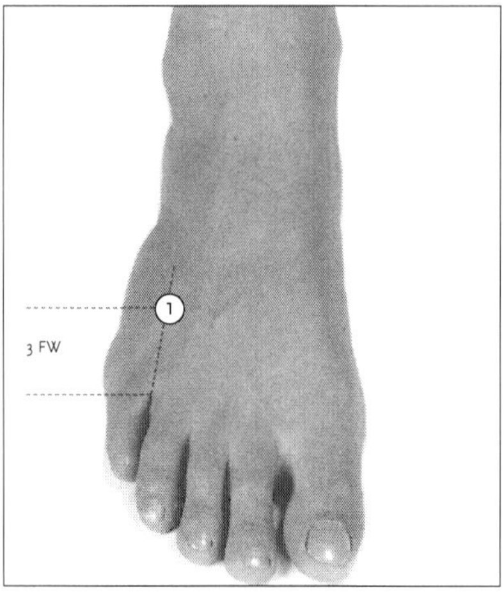

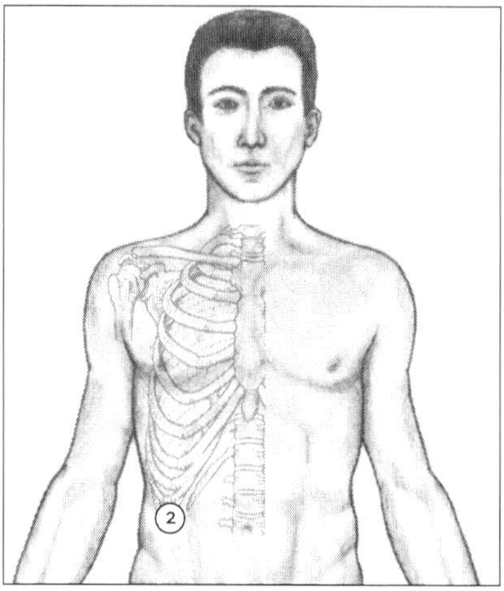

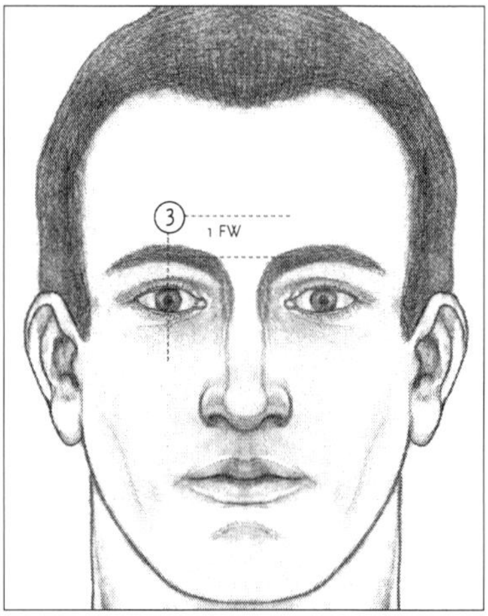

73 Gallbladder complaints

1 = GB 41, halfway between the top of the outer ankle and the webbing between the 4th and 5th toe ....yellow
2 = LV 13: at the end of the ribcage, on the tip of the 11th rib ..yellow
3 = GB 14: 1 FW above the eyebrow on a vertical line above the pupil (when looking straight ahead) ....yellow

All three points are treated only on the right side of the body.

Roberta suffers from hot flashes, sleeping disorders and lately belly aches – a nagging pain on the right side of the belly and pain at the right side of the neck. If someone says: 'I have neck problems', my first question always is: 'Right side or left side?' According to Peter Mandel the right side is connected with the gallbladder. I asked her to rub the zones at home with the esogetic herbal oil as described. After a week the complaints were less severe. She was also happy to report that the hot flashes were less and her sleep had improved.

Small and large intestine

The small intestine begins at the stomach and can be up to 6 meters long. In this long tract the main nutrients are separated and absorbed by the body. The remaining material that cannot be processed in the small intestine ends up in the large intestine, where other nutrients are digested and absorbed. The roughage finally leaves the body through the rectum. The digestive system is long and complications are likely to occur.

The intestines are of great importance to the entire lymphatic system. The lymph drainage from the head is connected to the intestines. If the lymph in the head isn't functioning properly and the waste materials from the head are not transported down to the belly, the intestines will also be affected.

The intestines are also connected to certain emotions, e.g.
- Susceptibility to sadness
- Having difficulty to let go
- Transparency, being permeable, influencing others or rather being suggestible and compliant
- Inability to indicate one's limits, overstepping one's limits
- Creativity, being creative or rather the inability to express one's creativity
- Inspiration, surrender

If these are actual themes in your life, you may also suffer from any of the following symptoms:
- Intestinal colic
- Gas or flatulence in the large intestine

- Irritable bowels
- Diarrhea or constipation

The following treatments will be helpful and don't take much time. You may notice that also the emotional issues that are related to the intestines start dissolving when you apply these treatments regularly.

LARGE INTESTINE

Location of the points and sequence of treatment:

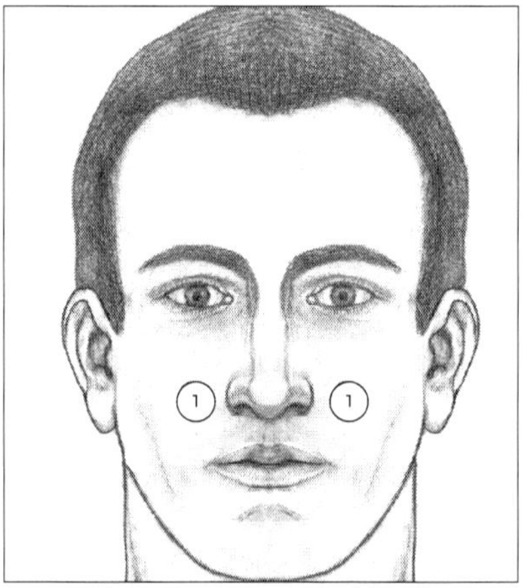

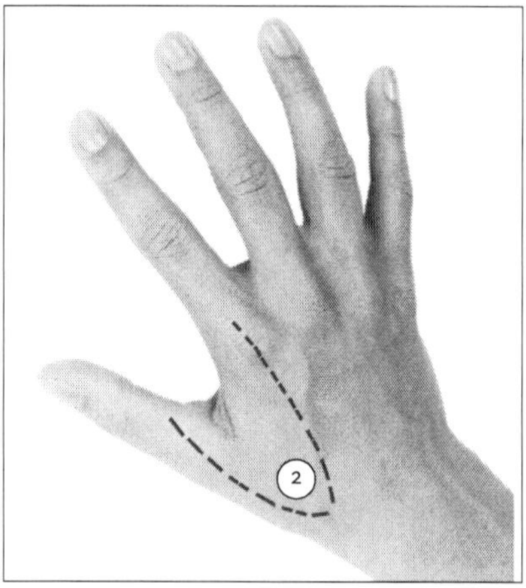

74 Large intestine treatment

1 = Points on the face, first on the left, then on the right ....red
2 = Points on the hands, first on the left, then on the right ...green

Location:
Middle of the maxillary sinus – follow the center of the eye downwards, the point lies on the lower edge of the cheekbone.
LI 4: at the highest point of the webbing between thumb and index finger, on both sides. This point is sensitive to pressure for most people. Don't treat this point if pregnant.

This treatment works on the sinuses as well as on the large intestine. It stimulates both of these lymphatic systems. The two points of the sinuses are combined with the acupuncture LI 4.

IRRITABLE BOWELS

This treatment works well when the intestines are irritated – the symptoms may be colic, flatulence, diarrhea or constipation, belly aches caused by stress, fear of examinations or any other emotional cause. Whoever has been diagnosed with 'irritable bowel syndrome' can give themselves this treatment daily. After the complaints have subsided, the treatment can still be repeated twice a week and eventually once a week.

1ST STEP COORDINATION 1

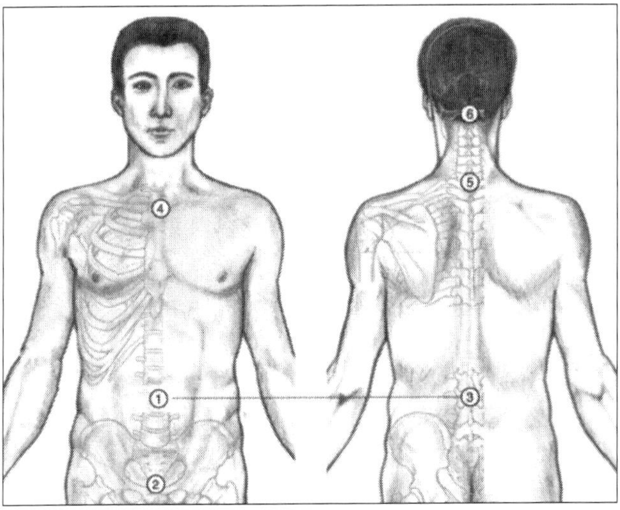

75 1st step: Irritable bowels – coordination 1

Location of the points and sequence of treatment:

1 = CV 8, the navel .... green
2 = CV 3, about 2 FW above the pubic bone, on the middle line .... orange
3 = On the back, on the spine, at the level of the navel .... violet
4 = CV 22, just under the throat, on the upper edge of the sternum in the hollow of the throat .... yellow
5 = GV 14, under the protuberance of the 7th cervical vertebra. When you feel along your neck, you find this cervical vertebra, that sticks out a bit .... red

6 = GV 16, at the back of the head, in the hollow between the scull and the first cervical vertebra................................blue

All points are treated 30 seconds.

2ND STEP AGGRESSIVE ZONES

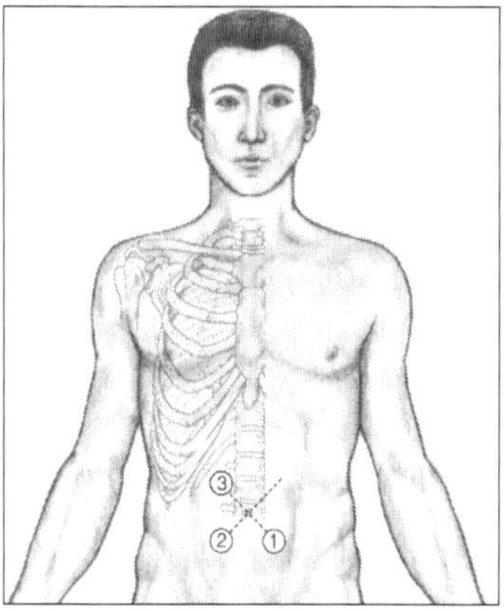

76 2nd step: Irritable bowels – aggressive zones

1-3 = Aggressive zones ....green

Location: on a diagonal line 2 FW up from the navel, down, left and right.

We treat three of these four zones: the lower point on the left, the lower point on the right and the upper point on the right – in this sequence.

These aggressive zones, situated around the navel, form the lymph triangle that activates the flow of lymph in the belly. By treating these zones we stimulate the activity of the small and large intestine.

Peter Mandel calls them the aggressive zones, because the waste materials stored here can turn aggressive against us. By radiating them with green light we help the immune system to protect us against attacks from inside or outside.

This treatment can also be given if one suffers from pain in the lower back, especially in the early morning. It also helps to relax neck and shoulders.

3RD STEP

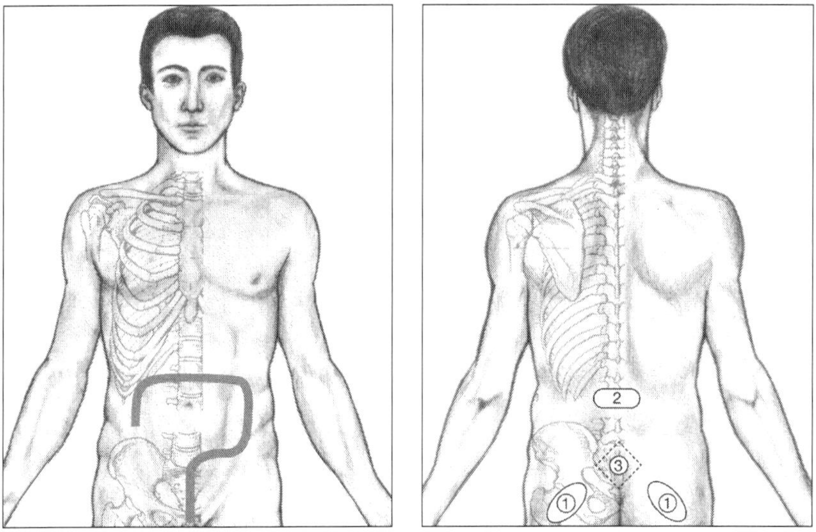

77 *3rd step: the figure of the intestine on the belly and the intestinal zones on the back*

Stroke the figure of the intestine .... yellow
Start on the right side of the belly, halfway between the pubic bone and the navel. Stroke up, then to the left and go down on the left side. Start again on the right side and repeat this five times.

1 = Intestinal zones on the buttocks: treat complementary .... yellow/violet
The more sensitive side is treated with violet, afterwards the less sensitive side is treated with yellow. Stroke the zones each for about 1 minute. If there are any painful areas in the zones, they can be treated for an extra 30 seconds.

2 = If this area is sensitive to pressure or if it has a rash .... violet
If this area is insensitive or cold .... yellow
Intestinal zone 2 is located on the spine at the highest lumbar vertebra, just below the ribcage.

3 = Intestinal zone 3: the sacrum .... orange
Stroke the entire zone for about 1 minute. This warms the lower body and the pelvis.

These intestinal zones on the buttocks can also be treated with the esogetic herbal oil. Especially if there are protracted intestinal complaints this is a very effective method of treatment. The gluteus maximus is painful for most people with intestinal complaints.

The ellipse of the deep subconscious

In the area of the 7th cervical vertebra Peter Mandel has located an important zone, which he called the zone of the deep subconscious. All that happens in our lives is recorded here, especially the events that have not been processed yet. Here all our unfinished emotional issues that we carry throughout our entire life are stored. This zone is the area where we carry our personal burden, our own cross, and here our development is slowed down. We cannot walk straight anymore, we are too heavily burdened. The cross we have created for ourselves becomes heavier all the time. Peter Mandel advises us: Do not carry what doesn't need to be carried!

We can lighten our burdens in life by giving extra attention to this area and by treating it preventively. The treatment of this ellipse has also proved to be a good remedy for complaints of the large and small intestine through the principle of the inverted man (as above, so below – up and down, front and back mirror each other). The principle of the inverted man has been explained in chapter 2.

In my practice I notice that clients who have been treated with this ellipse regularly, go through life with less burdens, breathe more deeply and feel more free. It is always good to give this treatment in case of tension in the shoulders, especially around the 7th cervical vertebra. Often reactions come within seconds during this treatment, as we contact deeper layers of consciousness.

ELLIPSE OF THE DEEP SUBCONSCIOUS

Location of the ellipse:
The top lies between the 6th and 7th cervical vertebra (C6 and C7). C7 is the vertebra that sticks out a bit. The lowest point is the spinal protuberance of the 2nd thoracic vertebra (Th2). The outer points are

located at 2 FW from the center to the left and the right. The ellipse is formed by connecting these four points.

The treatment of the ellipse consists of two parts.

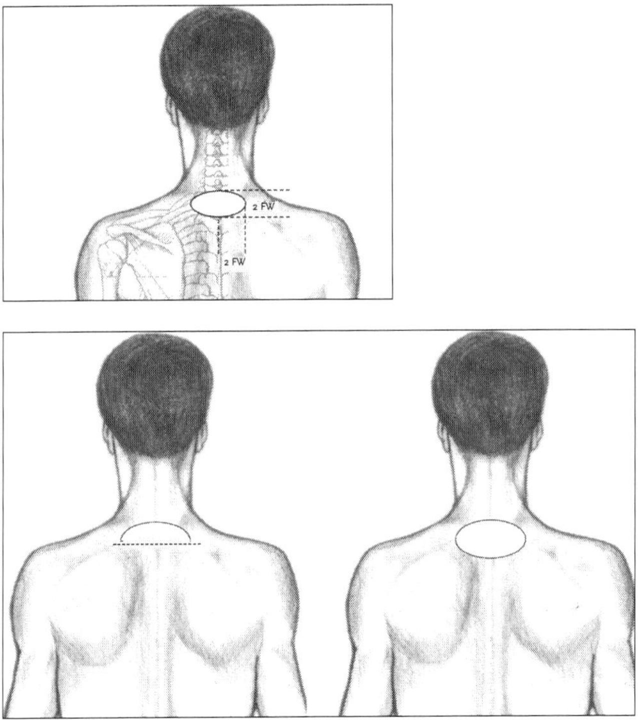

78 Ellipse of the deep subconscious

1ST STEP

Stroke the upper curve of the ellipse ....turquoise
Start the treatment at the upper part of the ellipse and stroke this curve for about 1 minute back and forth – in total about five times back and forth. If the body gives a signal by experiencing pressure, pain or an emotional reaction, it is best to wait for a moment and then continue. If the reactions do not subside, stop the treatment and wait till the next day before continuing the treatment. Afterwards the entire zone may be given a short massage and rubbed with three to five drops of esogetic herbal oil.

2ND STEP

Treatment of the entire ellipse..turquoise
After possible reactions during the 1st step have subsided one can continue with the 2nd step. Now we stroke the entire ellipse, first five times clockwise followed by five times anti-clockwise. If unpleasant reactions occur, change direction – usually the reactions stop immediately. If not, stop the treatment and repeat it after a few days, starting with the 1st step and followed by the 2nd step.

Listening to the CD Psychosomatic Balance has a beneficial effect in combination with this treatment.

All treatments described in this chapter can also be given to children.

> *Andrew came to me because of his belly complaints. The physicians he consulted could not find any specific cause for his complaints and labeled it irritable bowel syndrome. He also suffered from pain in neck and shoulders. He told me he could remember very little about his childhood. That gave me the indication to treat him with this ellipse of the deep subconscious. During the stroking of the ellipse with turquoise he started to get quite emotional without being able to explain why. His second appointment was a week later and then he told me he had had a dream about a house of which the windows and doors had been locked for a long time. Now they could be opened again! He also had experienced images and feelings connected with his childhood. One of them was the grief he had felt as a six-year old when his grandmother had died. I repeated this treatment a few times and his belly complaints diminished considerably.*

10

Conflict resolution

In this last chapter I would like to discuss in more detail the possible causes of disease. Looking at the genesis of an individual sickness, we usually encounter traumas and inner conflicts that have, to some extent, caused the ailments of this particular person. In this context it is important to realize that the cancer of patient X is not identical to the cancer of patient Y, even if they share the same diagnosis and lab test results. Why is this so? Because they each have their unique life history that is reflected in their bodies.

Regina was diagnosed with breast cancer three months after her son had died in a car accident. She could see that there was a connection between those two events and managed, after a short period of radiation therapy, to heal herself with natural remedies. She was willing to feel her grief and to process it.

It is up to each individual to discover what the inner conflict is that causes the sickness that has appeared in his or her life. There are as many causes as there are individuals and each sickness carries a message that wants to be heard and understood. The common denominator is the word 'conflict'. How to find this conflict and how to solve it – that is the theme of this chapter.

These conflicts are not the confrontations we have with others in our private lives or at work, but the inner conflicts that result when feeling and thinking give us conflicting messages. Your feeling may tell you that you need to change your job, but your practical mind tells you: 'Stop complaining, you need to earn a living'. Your inner voice tells you clearly that the relationship you are in is not good for you, but you fear the consequences of a divorce, you are convinced that a separation is just not done or not feasible. You know quite well that it is not a good idea to have so many drinks, but you are tempted again and again because you don't want to upset your friends. All those inner voices express a part of your truth and want to be heard. All aspects of your personality want to be respected, but if they do not get that respect, an inner conflict emerges. This inner tug-of-war consumes an enormous amount of energy, because you continuously need to silence one or more of these inner voices.

Another cause of conflict may be an experience in your childhood that is so horrible that you refuse to think about it – it is hidden so deeply that you hardly realize it is still there. This pressure of keeping a secret and repressing it, burdens the immune system. Over the years it becomes weaker and a sickness may be the result.

'Illness begins inside us in very small ways,' Peter Mandel says. 'Conflicts leave traces, no matter how deeply we manage to bury them. Like the lime deposits that, drop by drop, eventually produce stalagmites in caves, these traces accumulate; they get stronger and stronger until, in the end, an organ gets sick. And then the person enters into the arena of official medical care, and a stomach ulcer or diabetes or a swollen liver is diagnosed and treated. But they are only treating the last link in a very long chain.'

Mandel has set himself the task to find the cause of the sickness, together with the patient. He uses colorpuncture to literally shine the light on the dormant conflict to let it emerge, to let it come into the conscious mind. It can then be faced and eventually it will dissolve. Light and color introduce the correct information in the body and the mind, which can resolve the traumas that have led to a 'faulty programming'. These unresolved traumas can be compared to a computer virus which disturbs the software and causes the programs to malfunction.

After the trauma or the pain resulting from the past has come to light, the body needs to be given an impulse to become active. The energy needs to flow again. Only when the energy flow is restored the body can start regulating itself again. According to Peter Mandel this is the only way to bring stuck and rigid bodily systems back into flow.

Mandel has developed a series of treatments using light and color for this purpose. They are called 'Conflict Resolution'. In this book these treatments are not described, because they may only be applied by trained and certified colorpuncture therapists or be given as homework to their clients under their guidance.

However, there is a sound version of this Conflict Resolution treatment available on CDs. Ludovika Helm and Kay Korten-Helm have transferred these treatments into sound structures that are available for home treatment.

The CD series Conflict Resolution consists of 4 CDs and offers a way of treatment, not only in case of sickness, but also as a prevention whenever repetitive, restricting life patterns occur in your life. It offers an excellent aid to conquer difficult situations in life and supports the recognition and dissolution of potentially pathogenic patterns and conflicts. It ultimately is an aid to create a happy, vital and creative life.

The titles of the four CDs indicate the different phases of this audio therapy.

The first CD is called 'Cone of Memory'. By allowing memories to surface and by watching them from a certain distance, burdensome patterns are seen and released.

The second CD has the title: 'Resolution of blockages'.

The third CD is called: 'Letting Go'.

After passing these three phases the energy can increase. Therefore the fourth CD has the title 'Energy Increase'.

The four CDs have a logical sequence. Blockages cannot be removed before the cause has surfaced in our memory, which happens in the subconscious realm where they lie hidden. They can only be released once we have found the solution. Increase of energy is only possible when we remember the hidden conflicts, recognize the resulting blockages and let go of them.

A patient suffering from liver cancer came to my practice for treatment. His medical care program was finished – he only received medication and treatments to make the pain bearable. He was quite a young man, had just turned forty and had two young children – too young to die and still very much involved in life. He was not ready to leave and still had so many projects to finish. I gave him the colorpuncture treatment Conflict Resolution several times. It helped him to relax. In fact, he experienced for the first time how it feels to be relaxed. He didn't fall asleep, but went into a deep state of inner peace and relaxation, which was a real gift for him. His inner conflict was related to his need to perform and achieve. He was convinced that he could only perform under tension. Now he could allow relaxation to happen and saw that he could function very well from a relaxed state of mind. Such a treatment can offer a patient an extra lifespan, often months or years, in which insights and acceptance can result.

Lana also came for this conflict solving treatment. She had ovarian cancer and had been operated. She had received radiation therapy, chemotherapy and now refused further medical treatment. The initial prognosis was that she would live for another year. Five years later she was still alive with the help of alternative and additional treatments and her physical condition was reasonable. For one year Lana listened to the CD series Conflict Resolution and received the conflict solving colorpuncture treatments. She went through intense inner struggles, due to her past, her family, brothers and parents. After some time these inner struggles relented and she felt very grateful for that. She has passed away now, but she was calm and peaceful during the final stage of her life.

'As if a light has been switched on' is a remark I often hear from my clients after a treatment. That makes working with colorpuncture so fascinating for me. I notice how we become more conscious, more in touch with our inner core, with our path in life. The heaviness drops away and the sun shines for us once again. The light that we were born with is once more the central focal point in our lives and radiates in all colors of the rainbow.

This is my wish for all readers and users of this book:

good health and a life full of light, vitality and happiness.

Annex 1: List of treatments

Annex 2: List of points and meridians

Acupuncture points mentioned in this book
Alphabetical list of the meridians

Bladder meridian

UB 18: next to the protuberance of the 9th thoracic vertebra, 2 FW from the middle of the spine

UB 23: between L2 and L3 (lumbar vertebra 2 and 3), 2 FW from the middle of the spine

UB 31: in the upper hole of the sacrum, 2 FW next to the middle line, left and right

UB 37: in the middle of the back of the thigh

UB 40: in the middle of the back of the knee

UB 67: at the nail bed of the little toe, on the outside

Conception vessel meridian

CV 3: about 2 FW up from the edge of the pubic bone, on the middle line

CV 12: between the navel and the tip of the sternum

CV 14: 1 FW under the tip of the sternum

CV 17/18: in the middle of the sternum, between the top and the lower tip of the sternum

CV 22: under the throat, on the upper edge of the sternum in the hollow of the throat

Large intestine meridian

LI 4: at the highest point of the webbing between thumb and index finger, on both sides

Small intestine meridian

SI 11: in the center of the shoulder blade, 1 FW up from the line that connects the armpits

Gallbladder meridian

GB 14: 1 FW above the eyebrow on a vertical line up from the pupil (when looking straight ahead)

GB 25: at the free end of the 12th rib

GB 41: halfway between the top of the outer ankle and the webbing between the 4th and 5th toe

Governer vessel meridian

GV 2: at the beginning of the anal cleft

GV 9: under the protuberance of the 7th thoracic vertebra

GV 14: under the protuberance of the 7th cervical vertebra. When you feel along your neck, you find this cervical vertebra that sticks out a bit

GV 16: at the back of the head, in the hollow between the skull and the first cervical vertebra

GV 19: the point at the back of the head where the skull curves down. About 4 FW behind GV 20 on the middle line

GV 20: on the top of the head, in the middle, at the cross point of the horizontal and vertical line

GV 26: a little up from the center point between upper lip and the bottom of the nose

Liver meridian

LV 13: at the end of the ribcage, on the tip of the 11th rib

Lung meridian

LU 1: under the collarbone, about 6 FW to the side of the middle line of the body

LU 5: in the fold of the elbow, at the thumb side of the tendon in the fold of the elbow, left and right

LU 7: 2 FW under the first fold of the wrist

Lymph meridian (according to Voll)

Lymph 11: about 2 FW to the left and right of CV 22, in the corner between the collarbone and the muscle that is clearly visible when you turn your head

Stomach meridian

ST 25: 2 FW left and right of the navel

ST 27: 2 FW to the left and the right of the navel and 4 FW below it

ST 36: this point is found below and to the side of the knee on the outside of the leg. If you put the palm of your hand on your knee (left hand on left knee) and spread your fingers the ring finger lies on this point

ST 41: in the indentation of the foot, in the hollow

ST 45: on the cuticle of the 2nd toe, towards the 3rd toe

Spleen/pancreas meridian

SP 2: in front of the main joint of the big toe

SP 3: behind the main joint of the big toe

SP 4: 2 FW behind SP 3

SP 6: at the outer edge of the tibia, 4 FW above the inside of the ankle bone. Do not treat this point if pregnant!

Kidney meridian

KD 1: on the sole of the foot, between the 2nd and 3rd toe, in an indentation that is found when the toes are bent.

KD 25: between the 2nd and 3rd rib, 2 FW from the middle line

KD 26: between the 1st and 2nd rib, 2 FW from the middle line

KD 27: between the collar bone and the 1st rib, 2 FW from the middle line

Extra points

C4/C5: put your index finger halfway in the neck on the spine and bend the head backwards. The point lies in this fold on the spine.

C6: 6th cervical vertebra

C7: 7th cervical vertebra

Converter points for the kidneys: Between the 3rd and 4th rib. Find the middle of the collarbone and go 4 FW down

Kidney poles: in the angle of the 12th rib and the spinal protuberance of the first lumbar vertebra. Put your hands on your hips, place your thumbs against the lower ribs. Your thumbs will be on these points, which are always sensitive to pressure.

L2: 2nd lumbar vertebra

L3: 3rd lumbar vertebra

Th 2: 2nd thoracic vertebra

Th 8: 8th thoracic vertebra

Yin trang: between the eyebrows

Annex 3: Products

All products listed below can be ordered via the web shop of www.kleurenpunctuur.nl or www.esogetics.com

Light sets

These light sets are high quality products that have been developed under Peter Mandel's guidance for colorpuncture treatments. They are manufactured by instrument makers in Germany under supervision of Esogetics GmbH, the firm marketing all products for Esogetic holistic medicine.

Perlux P117

This light set contains one light pen, 7 glass rods in different spectral colors, a point locator probe and a spare bulb. The glass rods are handmade, the color is burned into the glass on one side of the rod and the top is pyramid shaped, concentrating the light on one point in order to effectively treat acupuncture points on the skin.

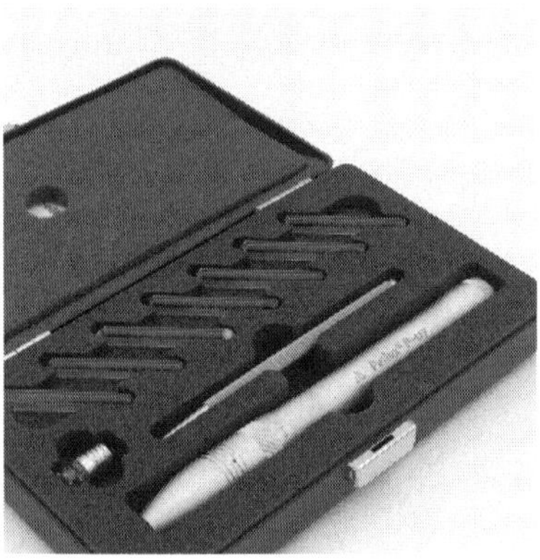

Perlux F333

This flat focus light set contains one light pen, 7 flat lenses in different spectral colors and a spare bulb. With this light set both points and zones on the skin can be treated. It is especially suited for those who want to treat themselves or their family members.

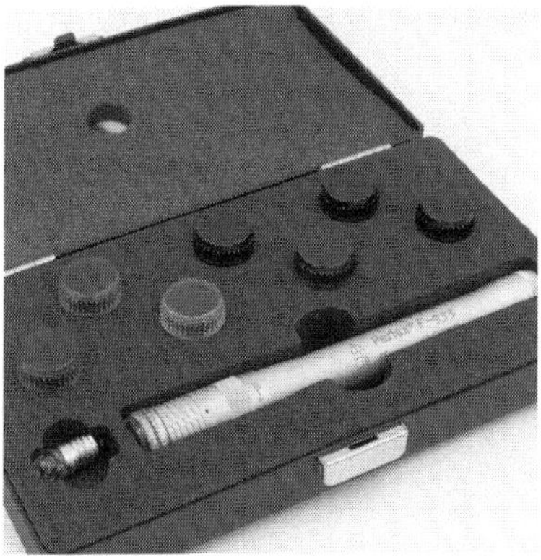

Perlux PF-450 Combination set

This is a combination of P117 and F333. It contains two light pens, 7 glass rods with pyramid focus, 7 flat lenses for treatment of zones, a point locator probe and a spare bulb.

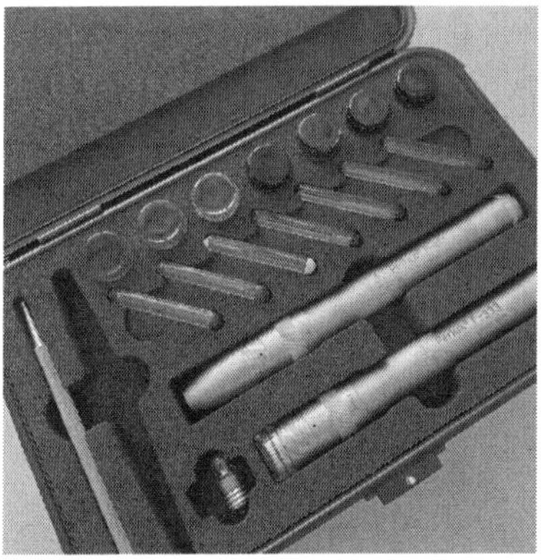

Information Energy Reflector

Peter Mandel has developed a small therapeutic instrument, which he calls an "Information-Energy-Reflector". The name ensues from the effect that this massage wand with the small crystal shows at all therapeutically relevant points on the skin. Meanwhile worldwide many people are treating themselves according to the zones and points that Peter Mandel has defined. The rounded point of the wand is intended for a localized massage of the point, and then the crystal is applied to the zone after a brief point massage of 10 – 15 seconds. All known reflex zones can be treated with the Information-Energy-Reflector. Experience the fascinating effect of the "Information-Energy-Reflector".

Available as a set in a case with the Information-Energy-Reflector and Peter Mandel's book The Matrix Reflectors".

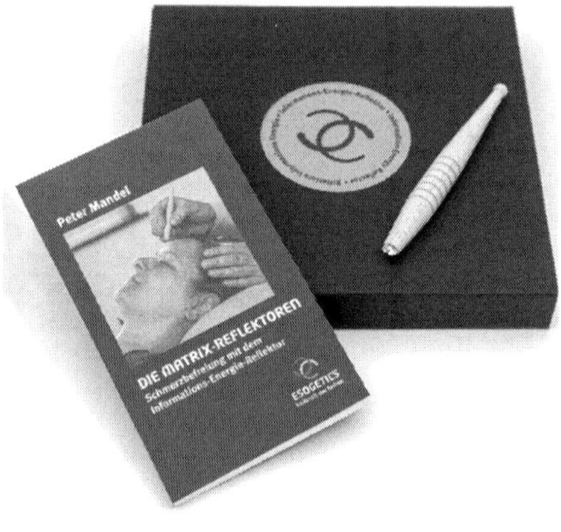

Esogetic herbal oil Relax

It is a well-known fact that essential oils have a stimulating effect. For thousands of years it is also known that stimulating certain reflex zones on the body by pressure point massage or acupuncture is very effective. By applying essential oils on the skin both methods are combined.

The esogetic herbal oil Relax is a mixture of various aromatic essential oils. It can be applied for treating a common cold, headache, stiff joints, muscle aches and painful limbs. When this oil is used on certain zones of the skin it activates dream activity, which is important to obtain a healthy, deep sleep, and helps us to be rested and start the day fresh. It promotes both physical and mental health.

The esogetic herbal oil contains extracts of several medicinal herbs, such as juniper, carnation, cinnamon, caraway, mountain pine, cedar, lavender, peppermint, rosemary, anise and eucalyptus.

In the book by Peter Mandel, *Dream Yourself Free! Activation of Dreams with Symbols*, you find many tips for the use of the esogetic herbal oil.

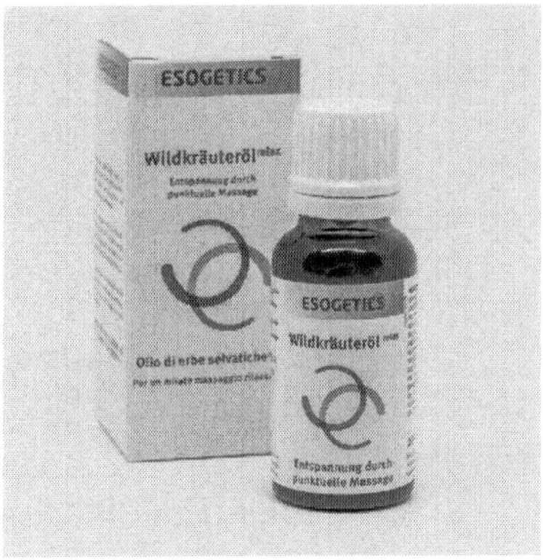

Sleep yourself fit

Sleep yourself fit with color, sound and herbal oil by Peter Mandel, adapted by Praveeta Timmerman.

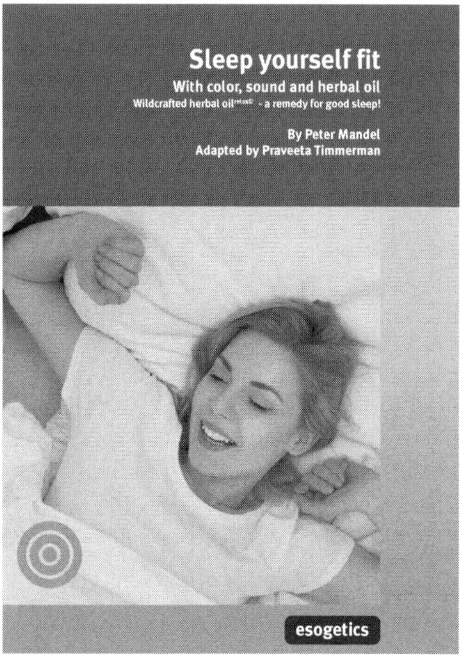

Sleep yourself fit! Yes, that is certainly possible if you follow the practical suggestions given in this book.

It gives you a clear how-to-do guide for the use of the wildcrafted herbal oil Relax as a remedy for good sleep. The book includes a section on the properties and qualities of this herbal oil, a section on how to promote dream activity as a means to improve your sleep and wake up fresh in the morning.

There is also a chapter on Color-Sound therapy and how to use sound to increase your well-being and inner harmony.

Color-Sound therapy – the soul listens as well

We often feel a subconscious longing for a type of music that helps us to regain our inner balance. Quiet sounds slow down the heart rate, promote relaxation and lower the blood pressure. Even sequences of tones with a high redundancy resolve tensions and reduce aggression and fear. While listening we enter a state of deep relaxation, the heart rate lowers and the respiration deepens and slows down.

Ludovika Helm and Kay Korten, both music scientists, have found a way to convert the colors used in Peter Mandel's colorpuncture into sound frequencies and Color-Sound therapy was born. The human ear can hear up to 1500 tones. They had to find the right sound combinations to reach the brain through our hearing. In the brain the vibrations resonate and influence the areas where dissonant frequencies have occurred. The harmonizing information is introduced by sound vibrations.

The sound that is equivalent with the therapeutic color consists of several tones. Color-Sound therapy exclusively uses pure frequencies that give harmonizing impulses to the brain. This deliberate use of tones and sound combinations helps the listener to feel better, both physically and mentally. They have an important regulating influence on the chemical reactions in the body. An inner harmony happens automatically, without the need to mentally try to solve the problems.

Certain psychosomatic sicknesses can be influenced by a selection of tones. Our hearing therefore is more than our 7th sense – it offers great opportunities that can be used to improve our well-being.

Conflict Resolution, a set of 4 CDs
By listening to these CDs old inner conflicts can be brought to the surface and be resolved. This set offers an aid in times of hardship and helps us to break through restrictive, stuck patterns. The CDs have the following topics:

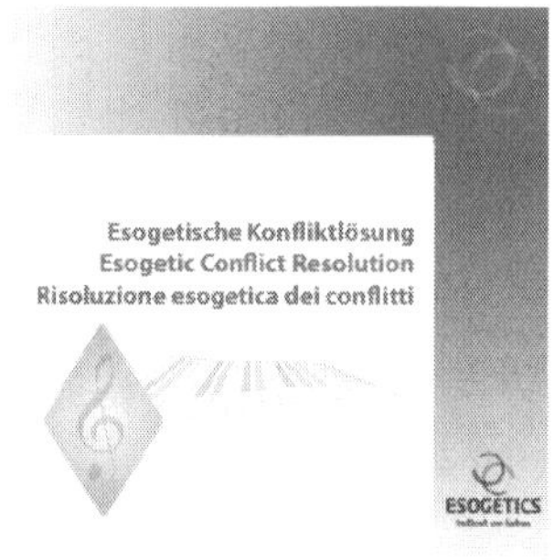

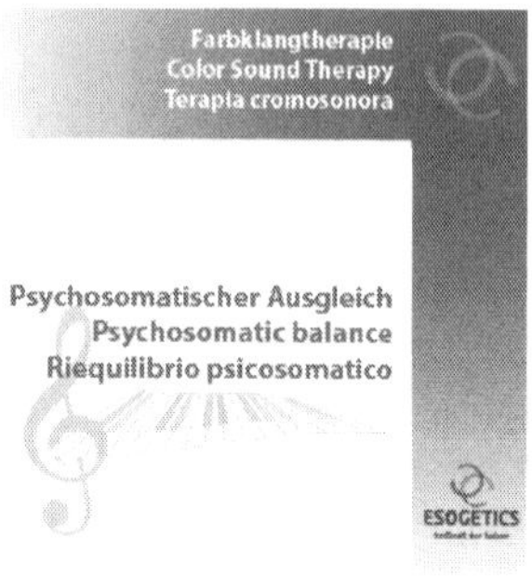

- Remembering
- Resolution of blockages
- Letting go
- Energy increase

One listens to one CD each day, in the sequence 1-4.

CD Psychosomatic Balance
The music tones on this CD restore the emotional and hormonal balance. Listening to this CD has helped many people with stress situations in school, at work or in private life. One can also listen to this CD in case of inner conflict, anger or in hectic times.

The CD contains two pieces of music, each of 20 minutes. As a start one can listen to one of the pieces daily and after a while once or twice weekly.

This CD is also useful for children and young adults.

The music tones on this CD regulate the energy body, especially in case of psychosomatic complaints, and help to digest the many impressions that we absorb each day. The effect of this music on the body and the coordination organs can be compared with a colorpuncture treatment.

CD Headaches/Migraine
Listening to this CD decreases the cramps in the brain and helps to prevent headaches. By regularly listening to this piece of 20 minutes can avoid the onset of a headache or a migraine and after a while the headaches will not occur anymore.

CD Sleeping Disorders
An aid to relax, this CD promotes a natural sleep.

Stress, problems, depressions and pain are the most common factors leading to sleeping disorders. The sounds on this CD help to resolve these, to harmonize and soothe overactivity in the brain. Most of these blockages will be removed, either consciously or unconsciously, making it easier to sleep. The sleep will be deeper and more restful.

In the beginning it is good to listen daily to this CD, after a while a few times a week will be sufficient. There are two pieces of music to choose from, each lasting 20 minutes.

CD Immune Activity
This CD supports the release of toxins and strengthens the immune system. The immunity against infections gets a boost and it also supports the emotional resilience. This sound therapy can effectively treat skin problems, flu and viral infections.

In the beginning it is advisable to listen daily to the music on this CD (20 minutes), later twice or thrice weekly will be sufficient. It is also suitable for children.

CD Concentration
The sounds on this CD increase the powers of concentration and improve the memory. Tiredness or pressure in the head are relieved. In the beginning it is good to listen daily to this CD, after a while a few times a week will be sufficient. Suitable for all ages, children as well as older persons.

CD Motivation

The sounds on this CD support the ability to learn. Listening to this CD will improve perception, memory, understanding and logical thinking. It also helps to process emotions and provides the motivation to lead the type of life that is right for you. Also suitable for children and young adults.

In the beginning it is advisable to listen daily to the music on this CD (20 minutes), later twice or thrice weekly will be sufficient. It is also suitable for children.

CD Totality: Spirit – Body –Soul

This set of 3 CDs harmonizes spirit, body and soul. The CD Spirit clears and regulates our perception through activating the thalamus, which controls all sensory perceptions and is regarded as the door to our consciousness. The CD Body helps to detoxify all bodily functions and improves the communication between the cells. The CD Soul harmonizes our emotions, stimulates inner stability and increases our vitality.

The CDs should be listened to in the sequence 1-3 on consecutive days. In the beginning twice a week, later once a week.

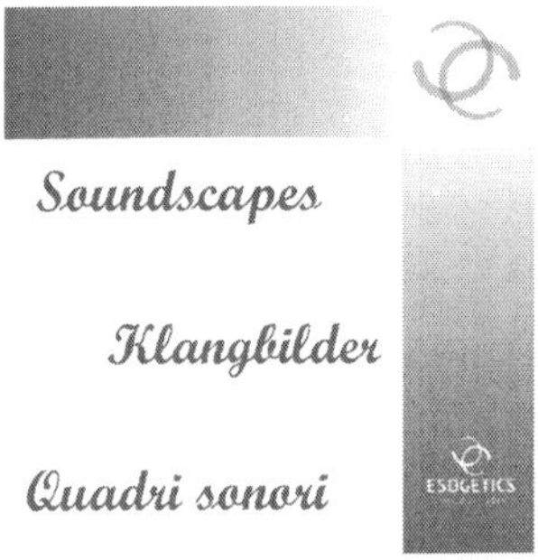

The Esogetic soundscapes have been developed according to exact mathematical and therapeutic parameters. The body is used as the key in this process, in order to be able to draw conclusions, from the recognition and interpretation of pain and illness, based on the actual content and tasks, thus on the entirely unique "program" of each individual person.

The special sound sequences and frequencies are also connected with the vibrations of the cell membrane. This is particularly important in relation to modern biology, the so-called epigenetics.

Listening to the nine "Esogetic Soundscapes" helps to stay healthy, but also to successfully treat some specific diseases, together with the necessary therapies.

No. 1: Balance
Supports the ability to let go of the old and to welcome the new, the precondition of serenity.

No. 2: Regeneration
Supports all processes dealing with change and reorientation.

No. 3: Self-Confidence
Serves as a "signpost" pointing the way to the essential human core.

No. 4: Vitality
This assists in accessing new insights and developing the strength to realize them.

No. 5: Self-Knowledge
Promotes the ability to recognize one's own powers and to use these to help remove mental barriers.

No. 6: Change
Reinforces the desire to become free of negative thoughts and to change behavioral patterns that could lead to problems.

No. 7: Reorientation
Shows possibilities to find purpose in life and to achieve one's life goals.

No. 8: Harmony
Supports us in leading a conscious, healthy and harmonious life.

No. 9: Completion
This compiles the most effective parts of soundscapes 1 to 8, as a repetition for refreshing all of the content previously conveyed.

Bibliography

Allanach, Jack
Colour me healing – Colorpuncture: A new Medicine of Light
Esogetics GmbH

Bailey, Alice
Esoteric Healing (A Treatise on the Seven Rays)
Verlag Lucis

Berendt, Joachim-Ernst
The World Is Sound: Nada Brahma: Music and the Landscape of Consciousness
Destiny Books, New Edition

Croke, Maohar
Energy Psychology using Light and Color
CreateSpace Independent Publishing Platform

Dethlefsen, Thorwald/Dahlke, Rüdiger
The Challenge of Fate
Coventure LTD

The Healing Power of Illness:
The Meaning of Symptoms and How to Interpret Them
Element Books Ltd

Gershon, Michael
The Second Brain: The Scientific Basis of Gut Instinct and a Groundbreaking New Understanding of Nervous Disorders of the Stomach and Intestines
Harper; 1 edition (October 7, 1998)

Leadbeater, C. W.
The Chakras (Quest Book)
Quest Books; 6th quest book printing edition (July 16, 2001)

Lipton, Bruce H.
The Biology of Belief: Unleashing the Power of Consciousness, Matter, & Miracles
Hay House; Revised edition (November 30, 2007)

Lipton, Bruce H./Bhaerman, Steve
Spontaneous Evolution: Our Positive Future and a Way to Get There From Here
Hay House; 3 edition (August 1, 2010)

Lommel, Pim van
Consciousness Beyond Life: The Science of the Near-Death Experience
HarperOne; Reprint edition (August 9, 2011)

Mandel, Peter
Compendium of the Ophtalmotropic Genetic Therapy – OGT
Esogetics GmbH

Dream Yourself Free! Activation of Dreams with Symbols
Esogetics GmbH

Sense and nonsense of sickness and pain
Esogetics GmbH

The Induction Therapy
Esogetics GmbH

The Playful I Ching – The oracle on the skin
Esogetics GmbH

Pagnamenta, Dr. med. Neeresh
Children in the Light – Colorpuncture for children
Esogetics GmbH

Pischinger, Alfred
The Extracellular Matrix and Ground Regulation: Basis for a Holistic Biological Medicine
North Atlantic Books; 1 edition (July 17, 2007)

Popp, Fritz A., Jiin-Ju Chang, Joachim Fritsch
Biophotons
Springer; 1998 edition (June 30, 1998)

Saint-Pierre, Gaston/Boater, Debbie
The Metamorphic Technique: Principles and Practice
Element Books Ltd (November 1991)

Schreiber, David Servan
The Instinct to Heal: Curing Depression, Anxiety and Stress Without Drugs and Without Talk Therapy Rodale Books (December 23, 2004)

Schönberger, Martin
I Ching and the Genetic Code: The Hidden Key to Life
Aurora Press (November 1, 1992)

Sheldrake, Rupert
The Science Delusion
Coronet; Airport/Export/Ireland ed edition (January 1, 2012)

Sheldrake, Rupert/McKenna, Terence/Abraham, Ralph
Chaos, Creativity, and Cosmic Consciousness
Park Street Press; New Edition of Trialogues at the Edge of the West edition (November 1, 2001)

Talbot, Michael
The Holographic Universe: The Revolutionary Theory of Reality
Harper Perennial; Reprint edition (September 6, 2011)

Taylor, Jeremy
Dream Work: Techniques for Discovering the Creative Power in Dreams
Paulist Press; annotated edition edition (January 1, 1983)

Walter Katya
Tao of Chaos: Merging East and West
Element Books Ltd (July 1996)

Wilber, Ken
The Spectrum of Consciousness (Quest Books)
Quest Books; 2nd edition (October 1, 1993)

Wilson Colin
Beyond the Occult: Twenty Years' Research into the Paranormal
Watkins (October 7, 2008)

List of Contents